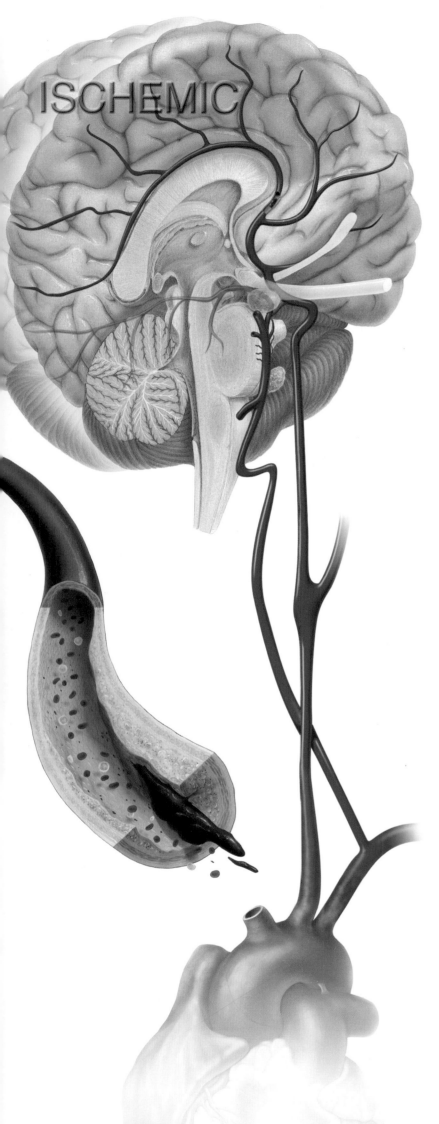

ISCHEMIC

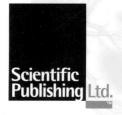

ISBN13: 978-1-932922-99-8   Item# PATH-25
Published in the United States by: Scientific Publishing Ltd. 129 Joey Drive, Elk Grove Village, IL 60007
Printed in Korea
Individual chart titles are available at www.scientificpublishing.com

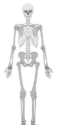

Understanding the Spine

Axial skeleton
Appendicular skeleton

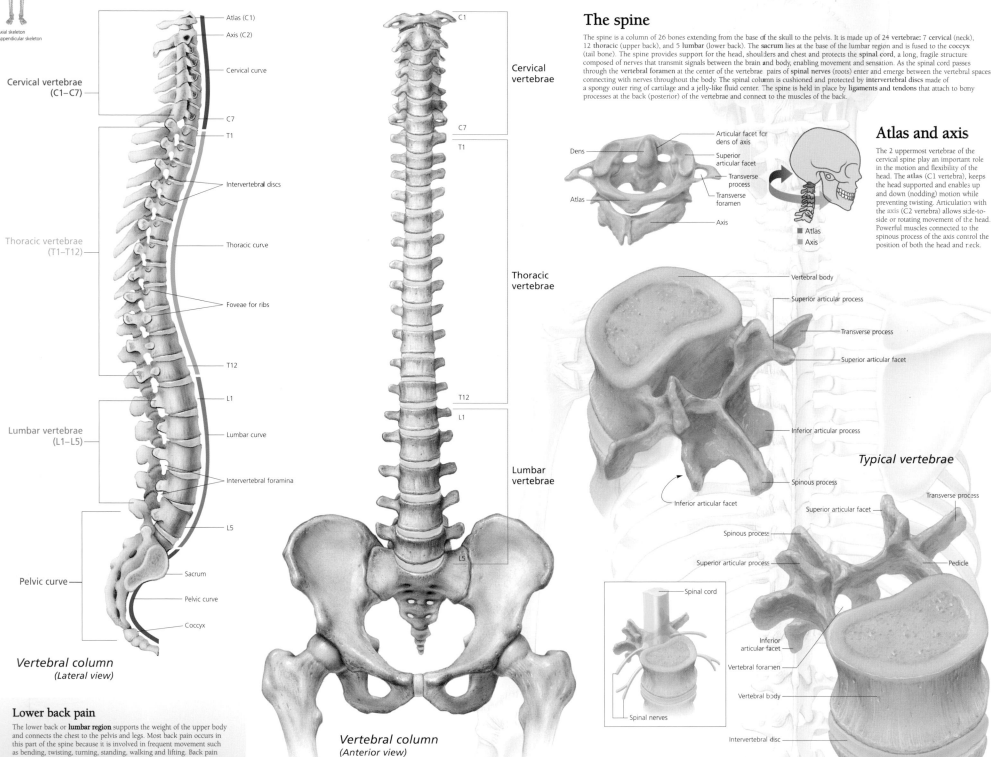

Cervical vertebrae (C1–C7)
- Atlas (C1)
- Axis (C2)
- Cervical curve
- C7
- T1

Thoracic vertebrae (T1–T12)
- Intervertebral discs
- Thoracic curve
- Foveae for ribs
- T12
- L1

Lumbar vertebrae (L1–L5)
- Lumbar curve
- Intervertebral foramina
- L5

- Pelvic curve
- Sacrum
- Pelvic curve
- Coccyx

Vertebral column (Lateral view)

- C1
- Cervical vertebrae
- C7
- T1
- Thoracic vertebrae
- T12
- L1
- Lumbar vertebrae
- L5

Vertebral column (Anterior view)

The spine

The spine is a column of 26 bones extending from the base of the skull to the pelvis. It is made up of 24 **vertebrae**: 7 cervical (neck), 12 thoracic (upper back), and 5 **lumbar** (lower back). The **sacrum** lies at the base of the lumbar region and is fused to the **coccyx** (tail bone). The spine provides support for the head, shoulders and chest and protects the **spinal cord**, a long, fragile structure composed of nerves that transmit signals between the brain and body, enabling movement and sensation. As the spinal cord passes through the **vertebral foramen** at the center of the vertebrae, pairs of **spinal nerves** (roots) enter and emerge between the vertebral spaces, connecting with nerves throughout the body. The spinal column is cushioned and protected by **intervertebral discs** made of a spongy outer ring of cartilage and a jelly-like fluid center. The spine is held in place by **ligaments and tendons** that attach to bony processes at the back (posterior) of the vertebrae and connect to the muscles of the back.

Atlas and axis

- Articular facet for dens of axis
- Dens
- Superior articular facet
- Transverse process
- Atlas
- Transverse foramen
- Axis

The 2 uppermost vertebrae of the cervical spine play an important role in the motion and flexibility of the head. The **atlas** (C1 vertebra), keeps the head supported and enables up and down (nodding) motion while preventing twisting. Articulation with the axis (C2 vertebra) allows side-to-side or rotating movement of the head. Powerful muscles connected to the spinous process of the axis control the position of both the head and neck.

- Atlas
- Axis

Typical vertebrae

- Vertebral body
- Superior articular process
- Transverse process
- Superior articular facet
- Inferior articular process
- Spinous process
- Inferior articular facet
- Transverse process
- Superior articular facet
- Superior articular process
- Pedicle
- Spinous process
- Inferior articular facet
- Vertebral foramen
- Vertebral body
- Intervertebral disc

- Spinal cord
- Spinal nerves

Lower back pain

The lower back or **lumbar region** supports the weight of the upper body and connects the chest to the pelvis and legs. Most back pain occurs in this part of the spine because it is involved in frequent movement such as bending, twisting, turning, standing, walking and lifting. Back pain is often classified as either **acute** (lasting from a few days to 3 months) or **chronic** (lasting 3 months or longer) and may range in severity from a dull ache to shooting or stabbing pain that limits motion, flexibility and/or the ability to stand upright. Because discs weaken with age, low back pain is usually age-related, occurring most frequently in adults through the mid-sixties.

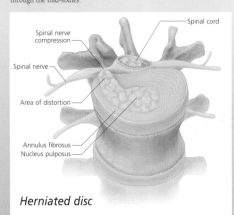

- Spinal cord
- Spinal nerve compression
- Spinal nerve
- Area of distortion
- Annulus fibrosus
- Nucleus pulposus

Herniated disc

Causes of lower back pain

Most acute lower back pain occurs as the result of stress on the muscles and ligaments that support the spine. A sedentary lifestyle and obesity also increase the risks of back injury and pain. Chronic back pain may be caused by underlying illness such as arthritis or depression. Treatment of back pain varies depending on cause and severity but may include heat or ice application, limited exercise, over-the-counter or prescription medications, or in extreme cases, surgery.

Typical causes of acute back pain include:
- Ruptured (herniated) disc
- Muscle strains or sprains
- Degenerative disc disease
- Spinal stenosis
- Sciatica
- Sacroiliitis

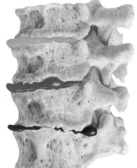

Lumbar vertebrae L1-4 with osteoarthritis (Lateral view)

Changes in joint shape cause painful compression of surrounding nerves

What is osteoarthritis?

Osteoarthritis (OA), also called **degenerative joint disease** or **osteoarthrosis**, has existed for centuries, occurring in many animals as well as humans. Currently, over 20 million people in the U.S. have OA. It is characterized by a gradual loss of cartilage and overgrowth of bone, often within only one or a few joints. Unlike other forms of arthritis, OA does not spread to other parts of the body. OA can occur in almost any movable joint but most commonly affects the spine, hips, knees, hands or feet.

Risk factors for OA

- Age (risk increases with age, affecting almost everyone over age 75)
- Family history of osteoarthritis
- Occupation that involves daily overworking of joints
- Injury to a joint
- Obesity

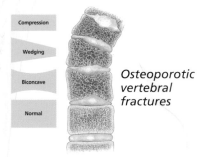

- Compression
- Wedging
- Biconcave
- Normal

Osteoporotic vertebral fractures

What is osteoporosis?

Osteoporosis is loss of bone mass due to an imbalance in the bone remodeling cycle. The lack of bone density causes instability and a greater likelihood of broken bones. Bones undergo change on a daily basis. Existing bone tissue is broken down and replaced by new tissue to provide bone mass. Under normal circumstances, the two distinct processes work together to provide a consistent bone mass. As people age, bone remodeling slows, but the tearing down of bone tissue continues at the same pace. The imbalance eventually creates a net loss in bone mass. This natural occurrence is worsened by not providing basic bone-building nutrients to the body such as calcium, proteins and vitamin D.

Risk factors for OP

- Post-menopausal women
- Ethnicity (Caucasian or Asian are at the highest risk)
- Family history of osteoporosis
- Eating disorders such as anorexia or bulimia
- Vigorous exercise program
- Overweight
- Alcoholism
- Thyroid disease
- Prolonged use of the anticoagulant heparin
- Males with reduced testosterone

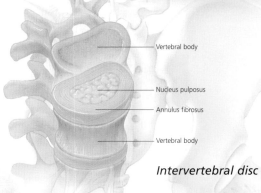

- Vertebral body
- Nucleus pulposus
- Annulus fibrosus
- Vertebral body

Intervertebral disc

Spinal deformities

In the normal spine, the inward curve of the lumbar spine is called **lordotic** and the outward curve of the thoracic spine is called **kyphotic**. Abnormal exaggeration of these curves or sideways curvature of the spine (**scoliosis**) may develop in children or adults with varying degrees of severity.

Lordosis or swayback is an excessive curvature of the lumbar spine. It may be congenital (present at birth) or caused by poor posture, neuromuscular disorders, hip problems, injury or infection. Exercise may stop the progression of the deformity.

Kyphosis is a thoracic spinal deformity that may be congenital or acquired as a result of other conditions, including Scheuermann's disease, which causes excessive curvature of the thoracic vertebrae. Symptoms may include unequal shoulder height, back pain, forward bending of the head and other complications. It may be treated with bracing or surgery.

Scoliosis commonly affects adolescents, particularly girls. Symptoms include side-to-side curvature of the upper or lower spine, unequal shoulder and hip height, sore or stiff back and other complications. Many cases remain mild. More severe cases may be treated by a brace or surgical bonding of the vertebrae.

PLATE 1

Understanding Arthritis

What is arthritis?

Arthritis is a general term used to describe any process that causes joint damage. There are more than 100 different types of arthritis, including **osteoarthritis** (also called degenerative arthritis or degenerative joint disease), **rheumatoid arthritis** and **gout**. Older adults are more frequently affected by arthritis, especially over the age of 75. Younger adults or even children may also develop the disease as a result of traumatic injuries, from wear and tear on joints, or from infections and immune system disorders. Arthritis may be located in the joints, the surrounding joint capsules, and the adjacent tissues. Some forms of arthritis also affect the skin, eyes, urinary system and digestive tract.

Three key diagnostic criteria help identify the specific type of arthritis: the presence of inflammation, the location of the affected joints and the number of joints involved. Diagnosis typically also includes blood tests, laboratory examination of fluid aspirated from swollen joints, x-rays and magnetic resonance imaging (MRI).

What are synovial joints?

A **joint** is any location in the body where two bones join and are held together by ligaments and other flexible structures. **Synovial joints** (i.e., hips, knees, ankles, shoulders, and wrists) contain specialized structures, including cartilage and synovial fluid. **Cartilage** is a smooth material that covers the ends of the bone joints to provide cushioning and allow movement. **Synovial fluid** helps to reduce friction during movement. Synovial joints may be affected by both osteoarthritis and rheumatoid arthritis.

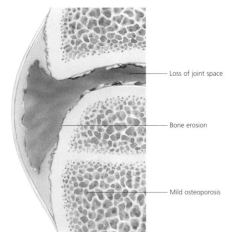

Synovial joint

Periosteum
Spongy bone
Compact bone
Synovial membrane
Articular cartilage
Synovial fluid
Joint capsule
Ligament
Muscle

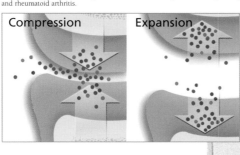

Compression **Expansion**

Exchange of nutrients

Unlike cartilage, the synovial membrane is loaded with blood vessels. Synovial fluid secreted by the synovial membrane is rich in nutrients from the blood. Since cartilage is like a dense sponge, repeated compression and expansion during and after joint movement circulates synovial membrane fluid throughout the cartilage, removing waste and delivering necessary nutrients.

What is rheumatoid arthritis?

Rheumatoid arthritis (RA) is a chronic, systemic inflammatory disease primarily affecting the synovial joints. For unknown reasons, the immune system attacks the linings (synovial membranes) of joints such as the hands, wrists, feet and knees. The onset is usually slow and often begins in small joints. A distinguishing characteristic of RA is that joints are affected in a symmetric pattern (i.e. both hands). As the disease advances, joints often become chronically inflamed, which leads to swelling, pain, stiffness and changes in joint mobility and function. Fluid and inflammatory cells accumulate in the synovial membrane to produce pannus, an invasive tissue that covers the surfaces of the joint's articular cartilage and erodes the cartilage, bone, ligaments and tendons. Continuing inflammation of the synovial membrane can eventually cause irreversible damage to the bones of the joint.

Characteristics of rheumatoid arthritis

1. Swollen joint capsule
2. Bone erosion
3. Cartilage erosion
4. Inflamed synovial membrane

Loss of joint space
Bone erosion
Mild osteoporosis

Joint with moderate rheumatoid arthritis

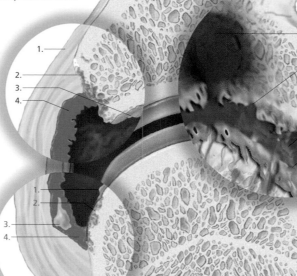

What is gout?

Gout is a form of inflammatory arthritis caused by the deposit of crystals in the joints and tendons. It commonly affects the feet, particularly the base of the first metatarsal joint (big toe), although it may also appear in the ankles, knees, wrists or elbows. The primary symptom is red, painful swelling around the affected joint, which limits range of motion. **Primary gout** is closely linked to an abnormal build-up of uric acid in the blood, a condition known as hyperuricemia. **Secondary gout** may develop due to an underlying disorder such as leukemia, kidney disease or enzyme abnormalities. Initial onset of gout is usually sudden and often occurs at night. After symptoms subside, months or years may pass between attacks. Recurring attacks can lead to the development of painful crystal deposits (tophi) and a more chronic, deforming type of arthritis.

Characteristics of gout

1. Cartilage erosion
2. Bone erosion
3. Sodium urate crystal
4. Inflamed synovium

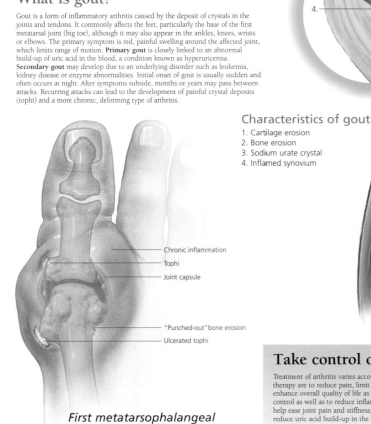

Chronic inflammation
Tophi
Joint capsule
"Punched-out" bone erosion
Ulcerated tophi

First metatarsophalangeal joint with gout (Tophi development)

Areas affected by arthritis

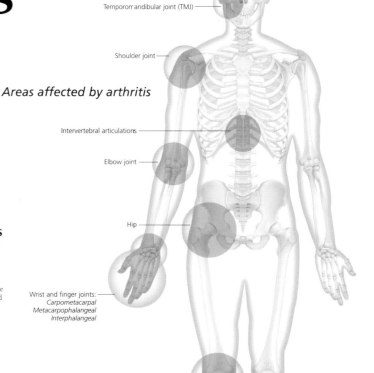

Temporomandibular joint (TMJ)
Shoulder joint
Intervertebral articulations
Elbow joint
Hip
Wrist and finger joints:
Carpometacarpal
Metacarpophalangeal
Interphalangeal
Knee
Foot and ankle joints:
Metatarsophalangeal

What is osteoarthritis?

Osteoarthritis (OA) is a degenerative joint disease characterized by loss of cartilage and overgrowth of bone (hypertrophy). It can occur in any movable joint. The two major types of OA include **primary osteoarthritis**, which typically develops slowly as a result of degeneration of cartilage in the joints of the fingers, hips, knees, and cervical (neck) or lumbar (lower back) spine. **Secondary osteoarthritis** can develop in joints as a result of trauma, chronic injury, disease or obesity. Osteoarthritis often begins slowly, characterized primarily by stiffness. As the disease progresses, a prominent symptom is joint pain, which is caused by the friction of bone against bone due to loss of cartilage. Over time, the joint may become stiff and decrease in mobility, causing the surrounding muscles to weaken. There is usually minimal swelling or fluid present.

Characteristics of osteoarthritis

1. Bone changes shape in response to friction, forming outgrowths of bone called osteophytes
2. Cyst formation
3. Superficial layer of exposed dead bone
4. Synovium absorbs fragments of deteriorating cartilage floating in synovial fluid and becomes thick and irritated
5. Damaged synovium and decreased use of joint due to pain can inhibit nutrient delivery to remaining cartilage
6. Cartilage erosion

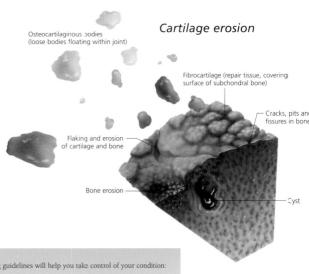

Cartilage erosion

Osteocartilaginous bodies (loose bodies floating within joint)
Fibrocartilage (repair tissue, covering surface of subchondral bone)
Cracks, pits and fissures in bone
Flaking and erosion of cartilage and bone
Bone erosion
Cyst

Take control of your arthritis

Treatment of arthritis varies according to the specific type of arthritis. In general, the goals of therapy are to reduce pain, limit progression of joint damage, improve range of motion, and enhance overall quality of life as much as possible. Medications may be required for pain control as well as to reduce inflammation. Exercise, physical therapy, and heat treatments can help ease joint pain and stiffness. Some arthritis-specific treatments include dietary changes to reduce uric acid build-up in the blood (gout); surgery to repair or replace damaged joints (osteoarthritis); and relaxation and stretching exercises to reduce articular inflammation (rheumatoid arthritis). A positive attitude can be beneficial in living successfully with arthritis.

For all types of arthritis, the following guidelines will help you take control of your condition:

- Educate yourself about arthritis
- Shed extra weight to decrease strain on your joints
- If necessary, use splints or braces to support affected joints
- Modify your living space to decrease strain on affected joints; for example, move frequently used items off high shelves
- Discuss potential medication side effects with your healthcare provider
- Work with your healthcare provider to determine an appropriate balance of exercise and rest
- Keep a daily record of activities, rest, medications, and any pain experienced to help determine what works best for you

PLATE 2

I Axial skeleton
II Appendicular skeleton

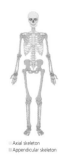
Axial skeleton
Appendicular skeleton

Understanding Osteoporosis

What is osteoporosis?

Osteoporosis is loss of bone mass due to an imbalance in the bone remodeling cycle. The lack of bone density causes instability and a greater likelihood of broken bones. Bones undergo a change on a daily basis. Existing bone tissue is broken down and replaced by new tissue to provide bone mass. Under normal circumstances, the two distinct processes work together to provide a consistent bone mass. As people age, bone remodeling slows, but the tearing down of bone tissue continues at the same pace. The imbalance eventually creates a net loss in bone mass. This natural occurrence is worsened by not providing basic bone-building nutrients to the body such as calcium, proteins and vitamin D.

What causes osteoporosis?

Osteoporosis is a common side effect of aging. Its severity is a function of risk factors, such as gender, genetics, diet and lifestyle. The highest risk group is post-menopausal women, who have lower levels of estrogen. (Estrogen carries calcium to bone tissue.) Younger women who experience amenorrhea (lack of menstrual periods) are at greater risk as well. Women who exercise excessively or have an eating disorder such as anorexia nervosa can develop osteoporosis earlier in life. At any age, whether male or female, a calcium-deficient diet would tend to increase the risk of osteoporosis.

Areas most affected by osteoporosis

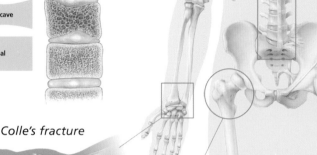

Bone density changes

Bone tissue density changes continually, because of the cycle of replenishing old with new tissue. From birth through adolescence, the cycle places heavier emphasis on building new tissue, resulting in a net increase in bone mass. As people reach their 20's and 30's, bone tissue is maintained at a healthy level because of the normal tissue formation cycle and a healthy diet and lifestyle. As women reach menopause, lack of estrogen production hinders the building of bone tissue. Men are affected to a lesser extent, but do experience net bone tissue loss.

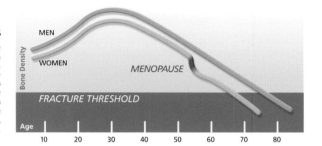

Osteoporotic vertebral fractures

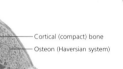

Compression
Wedging
Biconcave
Normal

The bone growth cycle
Formation and restoration

The process of bone remodeling continuously occurs throughout a person's life. Old bone is broken down and replaced by new bone. In osteoporosis, more bone is destroyed than is created, which results in a loss of bone mass.

1. The cycle begins on the trabecular plates (mature bone)
2. Activation of dormant cells, called osteoclast precursors, into bone breakdown cells called osteoclasts
3. Osteoclasts dissolve old bone and dig microscopic cavities
4. Bone-forming osteoblasts are attracted to the cavities, and begin filling them with a collagen matrix
5. Calcium & phosphorous crystals are added to the collagen matrix to strengthen & harden the bone

Colle's fracture

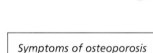

Radius

Osteoporotic bone

Cortical (compact) bone
Osteon (Haversian system)

Sites of hip fractures

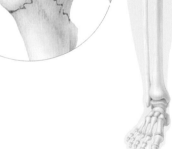

Femoral neck
Trochanteric

Trabecular (spongy) bone

Medullary cavity

Cortical (compact) bone
Osteon (Haversian system)

Periosteum

Trabecular (spongy) bone

Medullary cavity

Normal bone

Symptoms of osteoporosis

There are no early, unique or distinctive signs of osteoporosis, but if any of the following occur, a physician might diagnose the onset of osteoporosis.

- Back pain
- Development of a hunched back and abdominal protrusion
- Bone fractures resulting from an apparent minor trauma
- Reduction in height

Risk factors

- Post-menopause estrogen deficiency
- Ethnicity (Caucasian or Asian groups are at the highest risk)
- Family history of osteoporosis
- Eating disorders such as anorexia or bulimia
- Vigorous exercise program
- Overweight
- Alcoholism
- Thyroid disease
- Prolonged use of the anticoagulant heparin
- Males with reduced testosterone

Taking control of your osteoporosis

- Educate yourself about osteoporosis — it's easier to prevent than treat
- Maintain a calcium-rich diet — 1,000 mg to 1,200 mg per day
- Include vitamin D supplements in your diet
- Follow a reasonable exercise program
- Maintain a balanced posture to limit stress on the spine
- Take hormone replacement therapy, if directed by a physician

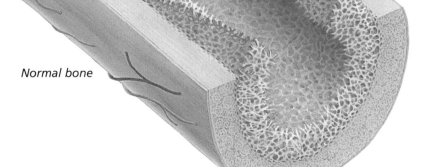

Effects of osteoporosis (progressive spinal deformity)

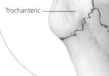

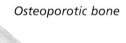

PLATE 3

Diseases of the Digestive System

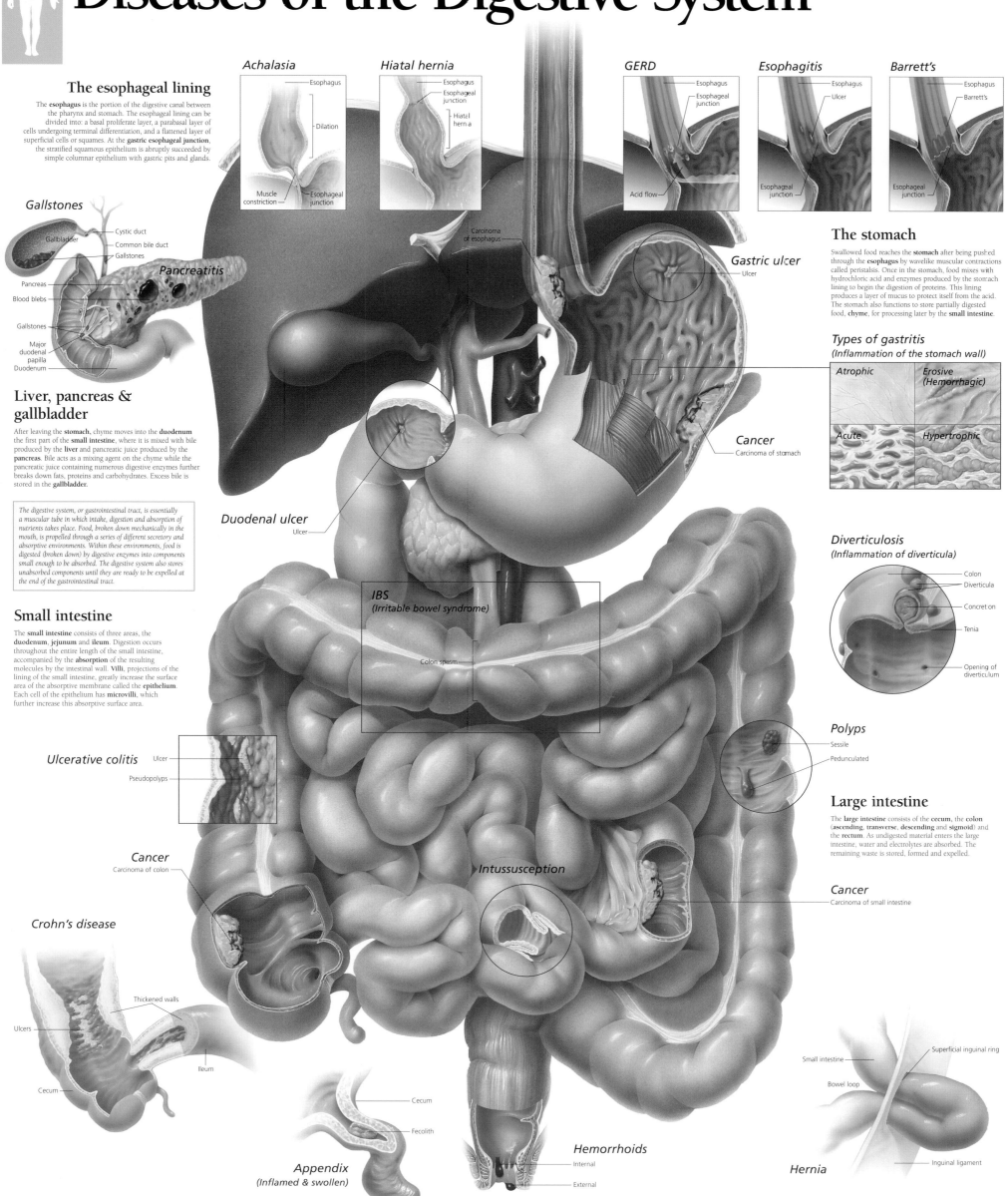

The esophageal lining

The **esophagus** is the portion of the digestive canal between the pharynx and stomach. The esophageal lining can be divided into: a basal proliferate layer, a parabasal layer of cells undergoing terminal differentiation, and a flattened layer of superficial cells or squames. At the **gastric esophageal junction**, the stratified squamous epithelium is abruptly succeeded by simple columnar epithelium with gastric pits and glands.

Achalasia
Esophagus
Dilation
Muscle constriction
Esophageal junction

Hiatal hernia
Esophagus
Esophageal junction
Hiatal hernia

GERD
Esophagus
Esophageal junction
Acid flow

Esophagitis
Esophagus
Ulcer
Esophageal junction

Barrett's
Esophagus
Barrett's
Esophageal junction

Gallstones
Gallbladder
Cystic duct
Common bile duct
Gallstones

Pancreatitis
Pancreas
Blood blebs
Gallstones
Major duodenal papilla
Duodenum

Liver, pancreas & gallbladder

After leaving the **stomach**, chyme moves into the **duodenum** the first part of the **small intestine**, where it is mixed with bile produced by the **liver** and pancreatic juice produced by the **pancreas**. Bile acts as a mixing agent on the chyme while the pancreatic juice containing numerous digestive enzymes further breaks down fats, proteins and carbohydrates. Excess bile is stored in the **gallbladder**.

The digestive system, or gastrointestinal tract, is essentially a muscular tube in which intake, digestion and absorption of nutrients takes place. Food, broken down mechanically in the mouth, is propelled through a series of different secretory and absorptive environments. Within these environments, food is digested (broken down) by digestive enzymes into components small enough to be absorbed. The digestive system also stores unabsorbed components until they are ready to be expelled at the end of the gastrointestinal tract.

Small intestine

The **small intestine** consists of three areas, the **duodenum, jejunum** and **ileum**. Digestion occurs throughout the entire length of the small intestine, accompanied by the **absorption** of the resulting molecules by the intestinal wall. **Villi**, projections of the lining of the small intestine, greatly increase the surface area of the absorptive membrane called the **epithelium**. Each cell of the epithelium has **microvilli**, which further increase this absorptive surface area.

The stomach

Swallowed food reaches the **stomach** after being pushed through the **esophagus** by wavelike muscular contractions called peristalsis. Once in the stomach, food mixes with hydrochloric acid and enzymes produced by the stomach lining to begin the digestion of proteins. This lining produces a layer of mucus to protect itself from the acid. The stomach also functions to store partially digested food, **chyme**, for processing later by the **small intestine**.

Carcinoma of esophagus

Gastric ulcer
Ulcer

Cancer
Carcinoma of stomach

Types of gastritis
(Inflammation of the stomach wall)

Atrophic	Erosive (Hemorrhagic)
Acute	Hypertrophic

Duodenal ulcer
Ulcer

Diverticulosis
(Inflammation of diverticula)
Colon
Diverticula
Concretion
Tenia
Opening of diverticulum

IBS
(Irritable bowel syndrome)
Colon spasm

Ulcerative colitis
Ulcer
Pseudopolyps

Polyps
Sessile
Pedunculated

Large intestine

The **large intestine** consists of the cecum, the **colon** (**ascending, transverse, descending** and **sigmoid**) and the **rectum**. As undigested material enters the large intestine, water and electrolytes are absorbed. The remaining waste is stored, formed and expelled.

Cancer
Carcinoma of colon

Crohn's disease
Thickened walls
Ulcers
Ileum
Cecum

Intussusception

Cancer
Carcinoma of small intestine

Appendix
(Inflamed & swollen)
Cecum
Fecolith

Hemorrhoids
Internal
External

Hernia
Superficial inguinal ring
Small intestine
Bowel loop
Inguinal ligament

PLATE 4

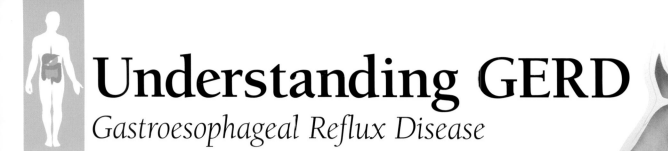

Understanding GERD
Gastroesophageal Reflux Disease

What is GERD?

GERD (gastroesophageal reflux disease) or **heartburn** is a frequent discomfort. About 1 in 10 adults has heartburn at least once a week; 1 in 3 has the problem at least once a month. Symptoms include a burning sensation in the chest that may start in the upper abdomen and radiate into the neck. Sour or bitter-tasting material is regurgitated into the throat and mouth, especially when lying down or sleeping. Continual chest discomfort after swallowing hard or liquid foods, inflammation of the esophagus, weight loss and vomiting of blood are symptoms of other problems often associated with GERD. Usually a description of symptoms will allow a physician to establish the diagnosis of heartburn.

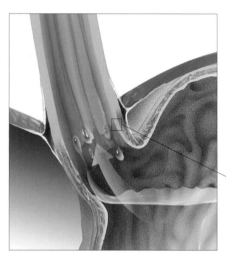

GERD
(Gastroesophageal Reflux Disease)

Under normal circumstances, food passes into the stomach from the esophagus and is prevented from traveling back up the esophagus by the lower esophageal sphincter, which remains tightly closed except when you swallow food. Sometimes, however, the sphincter muscle around the **gastric esophageal junction** becomes weakened and relaxes (opens), allowing acidic stomach contents to move back up the esophagus, producing the symptoms of heartburn.

Gastric esophageal junction

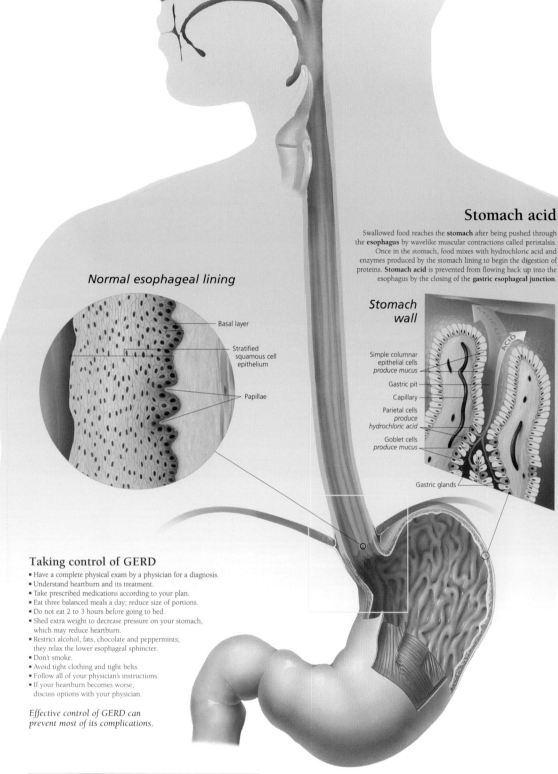

Stomach acid

Swallowed food reaches the **stomach** after being pushed through the **esophagus** by wavelike muscular contractions called peristalsis. Once in the stomach, food mixes with hydrochloric acid and enzymes produced by the stomach lining to begin the digestion of proteins. **Stomach acid** is prevented from flowing back up into the esophagus by the closing of the **gastric esophageal junction**.

Normal esophageal lining

- Basal layer
- Stratified squamous cell epithelium
- Papillae

Stomach wall

- Simple columnar epithelial cells *produce mucus*
- Gastric pit
- Capillary
- Parietal cells *produce hydrochloric acid*
- Goblet cells *produce mucus*
- Gastric glands

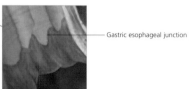

Esophageal lining with esophagitis

- Increased numbers of basal cells and thickened basal layer
- Ulcer
- Elongated papillae
- Vascularization of epithelium
- Epithelium

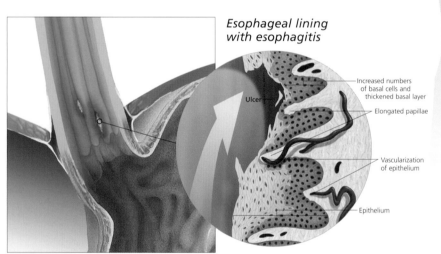

Esophagitis

When heartburn becomes more frequent, there is a chance of esophagitis, an irritation (inflammation) of the esophageal lining caused by stomach acid. If the esophagitis becomes severe, the result can be bleeding and difficulty in swallowing because of a constriction (stricture) of the esophagus. Some people with severe esophagitis develop Barrett's esophagus.

Taking control of GERD

- Have a complete physical exam by a physician for a diagnosis.
- Understand heartburn and its treatment.
- Take prescribed medications according to your plan.
- Eat three balanced meals a day; reduce size of portions.
- Do not eat 2 to 3 hours before going to bed.
- Shed extra weight to decrease pressure on your stomach, which may reduce heartburn.
- Restrict alcohol, fats, chocolate and peppermints; they relax the lower esophageal sphincter.
- Don't smoke.
- Avoid tight clothing and tight belts.
- Follow all of your physician's instructions.
- If your heartburn becomes worse, discuss options with your physician.

Effective control of GERD can prevent most of its complications.

Esophageal lining with Barrett's epithelium

- Esophagitis
- Abrupt change into abnormal specialized columnar epithelium in the esophagus

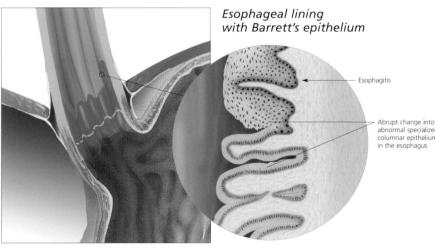

Barrett's esophagus

In addition to heartburn from a weakened lower esophageal sphincter, many other disorders can result in inflammation of your esophagus. Continual regurgitation of acid from the stomach may damage the normal skin-like lining of the esophagus, which is then replaced by a lining that resembles the lining of the stomach. This new lining usually can resist stomach acid, but inflammation at the upper end of the new lining may narrow (stricture) the interior passageway of the esophagus. Ulcers may occur in the new lining, and can bleed and perforate the esophageal wall. There is a slightly increased risk of cancer occurring in Barrett's esophagus.

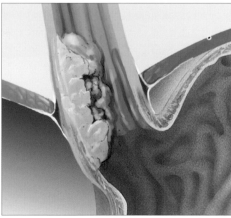

Cancer of the esophagus

Most tumors form in the middle or lower part of the esophagus. The principle symptom of an esophageal tumor is progressive difficulty in swallowing. Beginning with solid foods it will eventually become difficult even to swallow liquids. As the condition worsens, weight loss, the regurgitation of food and foul smelling breath probably will occur. Nearly 90 percent of esophageal tumors are malignant. Any difficulty in swallowing requires immediate attention from a physician for diagnostic tests.

Diet and medication

The ultimate goal of treating heartburn is to produce freedom from symptoms and prevent attacks. Improvements in lifestyle changes and diet alone may be enough to control GERD, especially in mild cases. Often, improvements in diet need to be combined with medication to control GERD. Due to the vast number of mechanisms in the body that affect the digestive system, there are several different types of medications. Your physician will determine which is best for you and may eventually suggest taking more than one.

Acid blockers decrease acid production in your stomach.

Proton Pump Inhibitors are a more powerful inhibitor of stomach acid production and relieves heartburn more effectively.

Surgery is rare and is only a viable solution for those with severe symptoms despite medication and lifestyle changes.

PLATE 5

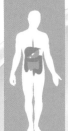

Understanding the Stomach

The digestive system

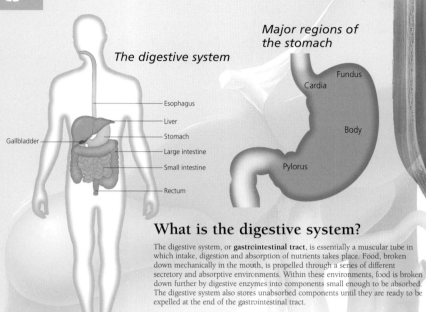

Major regions of the stomach

Esophagus

Cardia
Fundus

Body

Pylorus

The digestive system labels: Esophagus, Liver, Stomach, Large intestine, Small intestine, Rectum, Gallbladder

What is the digestive system?

The digestive system, or **gastrointestinal tract**, is essentially a muscular tube in which intake, digestion and absorption of nutrients takes place. Food, broken down mechanically in the mouth, is propelled through a series of different secretory and absorptive environments. Within these environments, food is broken down further by digestive enzymes into components small enough to be absorbed. The digestive system also stores unabsorbed components until they are ready to be expelled at the end of the gastrointestinal tract.

The stomach & digestion

Swallowed food reaches the stomach after being pushed through the esophagus by wavelike muscular contractions called **peristalsis**. Once in the stomach, food mixes with hydrochloric acid and enzymes produced by the stomach lining to begin the digestion of proteins. This lining produces a layer of mucus to protect itself from the acid. The stomach also functions to store partially digested food, **chyme**, for processing later by the small intestine.

Esophagus

Gastric esophageal junction

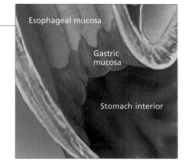

Esophageal mucosa

Gastric mucosa

Stomach interior

Fugae

Muscularis:
Oblique
Circular
Longitudinal

Mucosa

Submucosa

Serosa

Muscularis:
Oblique
Circular
Longitudinal

Stomach wall

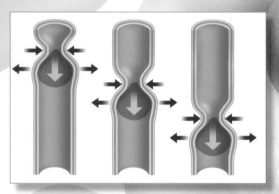

Peristaltic action

Waste material is moved through the digestive system by a series of muscle contractions called **peristalsis**. The contraction of the muscle behind the material moves it into the next section, where the muscle has relaxed.

What is a gastric ulcer?

Gastric ulcers, also known as peptic ulcers, are open areas in the lining of the gastrointestinal mucosa that have been injured by stomach acids and digestive enzymes (such as hydrochloric acid and pepsin). Two of the primary mechanisms believed to cause ulcers are non-steroidal anti-inflammatory medications (**NSAIDs**) and a bacteria known as **H. pylori**. These factors can disrupt the normal protective function of the mucosal lining of the stomach and increase the risk of damage from stomach acid. Other risk factors for developing ulcers include stress and smoking.

Gastric ulcers develop in the lining of the stomach and penetrate deeper into the mucosa than erosions. **Duodenal ulcers** occur only in the upper part of the small intestine.

Symptoms of gastric ulcers are known as dyspepsia, and may occur either chronically or occasionally. Dyspepsia frequently involves abdominal pain and discomfort, bloating, a feeling of fullness or an empty feeling in the stomach even after eating, nausea, and regurgitation. More severe ulcers can lead to complications such as hemorrhage and anemia.

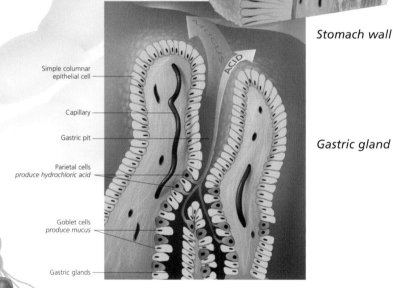

Simple columnar epithelial cell

Capillary

Gastric pit

Parietal cells *produce hydrochloric acid*

Goblet cells *produce mucus*

Gastric glands

Gastric gland

Gastric ulcer

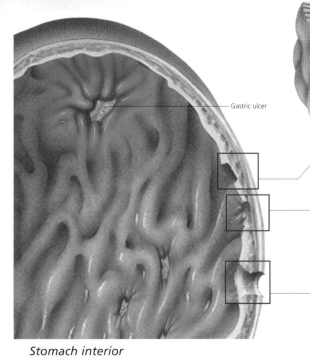

Stomach interior

Erosion

Ulcer

Helicobacter pylori bacteria

Perforated ulcer

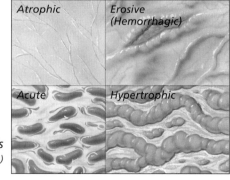

Atrophic | Erosive (Hemorrhagic)

Acute | Hypertrophic

Types of gastritis
(Inflammation of the gastric mucosa)

What is gastritis?

Gastritis is inflammation of the stomach lining (**gastric mucosa**). There are many factors that can cause gastritis, including infections, immune system disorders, certain kinds of drugs, excessive alcohol consumption and injuries. The Helicobacter pylori (*H. Pylori*) bacteria is a common cause of gastritis.

A sudden occurence is described as **acute gastritis**. In **erosive gastritis**, the stomach lining is inflamed and eroded; the condition commonly develops slowly. **Hypertrophic gastritis** is characterized by enlarged and thickened **rugae** (folds in the stomach lining), excessive mucus secretion and decreased acid secretion. **Atrophic gastritis** involves the disappearance of stomach folds, thinning of the stomach lining and loss of acid- and enzyme-producing cells.

PLATE 6

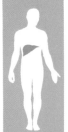

Understanding Hepatitis

Hepatitis B virus

Envelope
Double stranded DNA
Capsid

Hepatitis viruses vary in their specific characteristics but share a similar structure and infection process. A core of nucleic acid composed of DNA or RNA is surrounded by an outer protein shell with surface proteins or antigens that attach to the host cell. Once attached, viral nucleic acids are released into the host and replicate, generating new virus particles.

Surface proteins

Hepatitis B virus

Infection
is the first stage of hepatitis and occurs when the virus enters the body and invades the liver cells, prompting antibody response. Length of incubation time varies according to the type of virus.

Inflammation
occurs when the immune system responds to infection, causing injury or destruction in the infected liver cells. Inflammation can also result from exposure to drugs, alcohol and other substances.

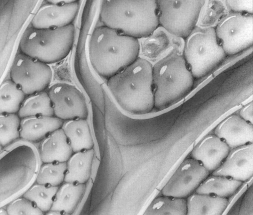

Fibrosis
is the growth of scar tissue following infection, inflammation or injury to the liver. Over time, scar tissue can inhibit normal liver function, including **blood processing** and **nutrient metabolism**.

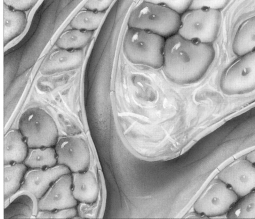

Cirrhosis
develops when a significant portion of the liver tissue has been progressively and irreversibly destroyed by injury or disease. Cirrhosis may result from **alcohol abuse**, chronic **viral liver disease**, or other causes and is often fatal.

What is hepatitis?

Hepatitis is an **inflammation** of the liver triggered by **infection** or **injury** and characterized by the destruction of significant numbers of liver cells. The severity of the disease depends on many factors, including the specific cause of the inflammation as well as any preexisting physical conditions. The symptoms vary widely according to the type of hepatitis and the duration of the inflammation (acute or chronic).

Acute hepatitis
The acute form of hepatitis evolves over a short period of time and resolves **within 6 months** (often 2 months or less). It may be caused by a variety of factors, including hepatitis viruses, medications, toxins and severe bacterial infections.

Chronic hepatitis
Acute hepatitis that persists for **more than 6 months** is called chronic hepatitis. There are many potential causes of chronic hepatitis, including infection by hepatitis viruses B and C. Chronic hepatitis can result in **persistent liver damage.**

Causes of hepatitis

Hepatitis can be caused by any substance or organism that damages the liver, including viruses, autoimmune disorders, alcohol, drugs and chemical toxins.

Viral hepatitis is the leading cause of liver disease in the United States. Symptoms of acute viral hepatitis may begin suddenly or develop over time. They often include nausea and vomiting, slight fever, fatigue, and pressure or pain in the upper right abdomen. Jaundice, dark-colored urine, joint aches, diarrhea and weight loss may also occur.

Autoimmune hepatitis occurs when the body's defense mechanisms attack the liver cells. It can be present in either chronic or acute form and may appear similar to viral hepatitis. Fatigue is the most common symptom, but other symptoms, ranging from mild to severe, can include enlarged liver, jaundice, and joint pain as well as itching and skin rashes. Autoimmune hepatitis is more common in women than men and may be associated with other autoimmune disorders.

Alcohol and drug hepatitis results from excessive or chronic alcohol use or following the consumption of certain drugs or medications. Symptoms include jaundice, fatigue and alterations in sense of taste and smell. **Alcoholic hepatitis** may produce symptoms ranging from mild flu-like characteristics to high fever and enlarged liver. If untreated, this condition can lead to **fatty liver, cirrhosis** or complete **liver failure. Toxic and drug-induced hepatitis** can be caused by a variety of prescription and over-the-counter medications as well as chemical agents and industrial toxins.

Nonalcoholic steatohepatitis can appear in patients with conditions including high cholesterol, diabetes and obesity who do not consume large amounts of alcohol. Symptoms are similar to alcohol-induced hepatitis.

Healthy cross section of liver lobule

Healthy Liver

Liver function

The liver performs more than 500 important functions, including its vital role as a portal between the digestive tract and the circulatory system. It is also an important source of **blood storage**. Approximately 1500 ml of blood flows through the liver per minute. As much as 13 percent of the body's total blood volume is usually contained in the liver, which can swell to hold even larger amounts of blood in response to injury or illness.

What is portal hypertension?

Portal hypertension is an increase in pressure in the portal vein that carries blood from the intestines, spleen and pancreas into the liver.

- In cirrhosis, damage from fibrosis can increase resistance in the portal vein, forcing blood to flow back towards the heart by the way of collateral vessels, instead of through the liver.
- Collateral vessels may develop to bypass the liver, connecting the portal vein directly to the lower portion of the esophagus.
- Swollen collateral vessels (esophageal varices) are fragile and can easily rupture, causing dangerous bleeding in the stomach.

Cross section of liver lobule with later stages of fibrosis, scar tissue

Contaminated food or water

Contact with infected blood

Alcohol use / Drug abuse

Sexual contact

Risk factors for hepatitis

- Exchange of bodily fluids with an infected person, especially through sexual contact or sex with multiple partners
- Consumption of contaminated water or food, including improperly cooked shellfish (HAV)
- Contact with infected blood through illicit drug use or occupational needle sticks
- Sharing razors, toothbrushes or other personal items that may contain blood
- Chronic or excessive alcohol use and drug abuse

Enlarged view of the liver lobule

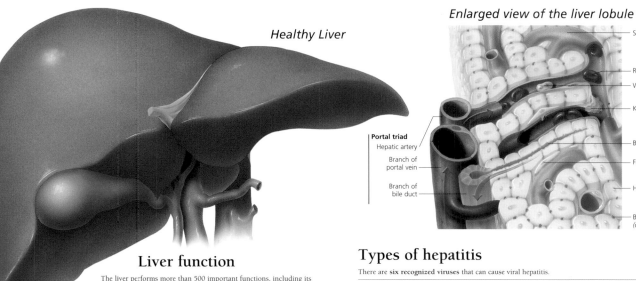

Sinusoid
Red blood cell
White blood cell
Kupffer cell
Bile canaliculi
Fat storing cell
Hepatocyte
Bile canaliculi (cross section)

Portal triad
Hepatic artery
Branch of portal vein
Branch of bile duct

Types of hepatitis

There are **six recognized viruses** that can cause viral hepatitis.

HAV
Hepatitis A Virus is an acute form of hepatitis virus that typically begins 2-6 weeks after infection. It is easily **spread** through **food or water** contaminated by the feces of an infected person or through **contaminated shellfish.** HAV usually requires no treatment and resolves over several weeks, although up to 15% of patients will have prolonged symptoms over a 6-9 month period. HAV can be prevented with **Hepatitis A vaccine.**

HBV
Hepatitis B Virus can cause both acute and chronic hepatitis. Symptoms appear within 1-6 months after infection and may be almost unnoticeable or produce a range of typical viral hepatitis symptoms lasting several weeks or months. HBV is extremely infectious and spreads through **body fluids, contaminated syringes and needles,** or transmission from mother to unborn child. HBV can be prevented with **Hepatitis B vaccine.**

HCV
Hepatitis C Virus causes both acute and chronic hepatitis; it is much more likely to produce **chronic liver disease** than Hepatitis B. Up to 80% of patients have no signs or symptoms of disease, which develop between 2 weeks and 6 months after infection. The chronic form can also develop without early symptoms, although liver damage is occurring. HCV is spread mainly through contact with **infected blood,** including IV drug use, needle sticks, and unprotected sexual contact. There is **no vaccine** for HCV.

HDV
Hepatitis D or Delta Virus occurs only in conjunction with Hepatitis B Virus and spreads through similar routes. Acute infection can be more severe if both viruses are present, although complete recovery usually occurs when infection with both viruses occurs simultaneously (**coinfection**). Patients who develop chronic Hepatitis B and are later infected with HDV (**superinfection**) experience more severe symptoms and are more likely to develop liver failure. HDV can be prevented with **Hepatitis B vaccine.**

HEV
Hepatitis E Virus produces acute hepatitis symptoms and is transmitted via ingestion. It is prevalent in developing countries where **water sources are contaminated** by human waste. Symptoms develop within 2-8 weeks and resolve completely within a month. Pregnant women are at greatest risk from severe illness or acute liver failure. There is **no vaccine for HEV.**

HGV
Hepatitis G Virus is a recently discovered viral form that may occur alone or in the presence of HBV or HCV. Little is known about the course of illness but research suggests that it is mild and short-term. HGV has also been identified in patients with chronic hepatitis. It is transmitted via the blood and there is **no vaccine.**

Diagnosis and treatment

Diagnosis is confirmed with clinical tests. Symptoms are also important but may not be present in all patients.

- *Blood tests* measure elevated **bilirubin** and **aminotransferase** levels and the presence of **antigens** and **antibodies** that develop during viral infection. After recovery, antibodies may remain, indicating previous infection. **Immune factors** (serum globulins) in the blood may help diagnose autoimmune hepatitis.
- *Liver biopsy* is required to confirm chronic hepatitis and determine the type and degree of damage from liver disease.
- *Other tests* such as ultrasound and liver/spleen scans may be used to diagnose cirrhosis.

Treatment varies depending on the type and severity of disease.

- Acute infections are typically treated with rest, a balanced diet, and abstinence from alcohol or certain medications that are metabolized in the liver.
- Chronic hepatitis treatment may include interferon and/or other specialized drugs.
- In liver failure, transplantation is the only treatment option.

PLATE 7

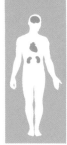

High Blood Pressure

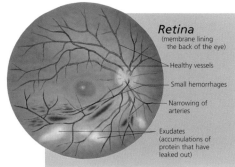

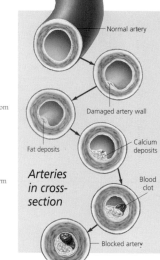

What is blood pressure?

Blood pressure is the force of circulating blood against the inner walls of the blood vessels. It is affected by:
- how hard the heart pumps
- the amount of blood in the body
- the diameter of the blood vessels

Generally, blood pressure increases when the heart pumps *harder*, the amount of blood in the body *increases* or the diameter of the blood vessels *decreases*.

Importance of pressure

Arterial blood carries essential materials such as oxygen and other nutrients to every cell in the body. Without an adequate supply of blood, organs and tissues cannot survive. Venous blood carries waste products away from the cells to be discarded. Both blood pressure and concentration must be within certain levels for this crucial exchange of nutrients and waste to occur. Fortunately, the body is armed with a web of complex mechanisms that monitor pressure and concentration and act to keep both within normal ranges.

Blood pressure forces blood into the tiny capillaries of the organs and contributes to the movement of nutrients out of the blood into the tissues.

In the venule, blood pressure is lower. Forces created by concentration differences cause waste products to return to the blood.

What is high blood pressure?

One out of five adults in the U.S.—more than 50 million people—has high blood pressure. The term **hypertension** is also used to describe this condition, but it does not refer to being anxious or tense. It occurs when blood is flowing through the vessels at a pressure that is too high for the long-term health of the blood vessels. Generally, a blood pressure of 140 over 90 or higher is considered unhealthy. Over time, vessel walls exposed to these levels of pressure become damaged. This damage can lead to serious health problems.

What causes high blood pressure?

Occasionally, high blood pressure is caused by a disease. This type is called **secondary hypertension**. Most people with high blood pressure have a type called **essential** or **primary hypertension**. Although there are many theories about primary hypertension, the exact cause is unknown. It is possible that several complex mechanisms are involved.

Risk factors

- Family history of high blood pressure
- Race (African Americans have the highest incidence)
- Age (risk increases with age)
- Obesity
- Sedentary lifestyle
- Diabetes mellitus

Measuring blood pressure

Blood pressure is a measurement consisting of a top number, **systolic pressure** (pressure when the heart is contracting), and a bottom number, **diastolic pressure** (pressure when the heart is resting). It is measured with a pressure cuff and sphygmomanometer. The cuff is placed around the upper arm and tightened until blood flow through the brachial artery is stopped. Pressure, read from the attached meter, is gradually decreased in the cuff while a stethoscope is used to listen to the brachial artery. Sounds heard in the artery indicate the blood pressure. Blood pressure can be measured this way because blood makes noise when its flow is restricted:

Artery is blocked: no movement of blood—*silence*

Systolic pressure, artery begins to open: blood flow is turbulent—*sounds are heard*

Diastolic pressure, artery is completely open: blood flows smoothly through the artery—*silence*

The average blood pressure reading of a healthy adult is approximately:

$$\frac{120}{80}$$

Salt and blood pressure

Blood pressure and blood concentration of salt are closely related. When you eat salty foods, blood concentration of salt goes up. Almost immediately, water is added to the blood by the kidneys so that blood concentration returns to normal. Additional water in the bloodstream elevates blood pressure. Blood pressure will stay elevated until the body is able to excrete the excess salt and water.

People with high blood pressure should watch their intake of salt. Although the exact role of salt is unknown, it is possible that some people with high blood pressure have a decreased ability to excrete it. Also, low salt intake may increase the effectiveness of medication.

Brachial artery

Pressure cuff

Stethoscope

Effects of high blood pressure

A person with high blood pressure usually has no symptoms until he or she has had it for quite some time and serious damage has occurred. For this reason, it is often called the "silent killer." Long-term damage from uncontrolled high blood pressure is often irreversible and can lead to an early death:

Retina
(membrane lining the back of the eye)
- Healthy vessels
- Small hemorrhages
- Narrowing of arteries
- Exudates (accumulations of protein that have leaked out)

Damage to the eyes

It is unusual for eye damage from high blood pressure to impair vision, but the retina provides a remarkably accurate assessment of overall damage to blood vessels. The small blood vessels in the retina are a good sample of all the blood vessels in the body and are easily inspected.

Damage to the brain

- **Stroke:** A portion of brain tissue dies when it is deprived of blood supply. This can happen when a bulging artery (called an **aneurysm**) ruptures or an artery becomes blocked by a blood clot or fat deposits.
- **Cerebrovascular insufficiency:** A series of mini-strokes occurs in the smaller vessels of the brain. Tiny arterioles bulge, then burst from high pressure or become blocked by small blood clots. There are no symptoms until damage accumulates over time.

Damage to blood vessels

Artery walls become damaged from high pressure. Fat accumulates and the walls thicken. Calcium is deposited in the fatty areas, "hardening" the arteries, making them unable to increase in size. Blood flow through the arteries decreases. Damaged artery walls may also cause blood clots to form which block the artery itself or break off and block arteries in other organs.

Arteries in cross-section
- Normal artery
- Damaged artery wall
- Fat deposits
- Calcium deposits
- Blood clot
- Blocked artery

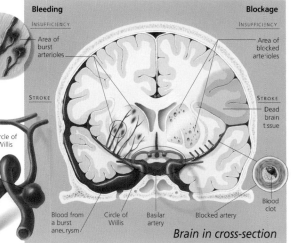

Bleeding — INSUFFICIENCY — Area of burst arterioles

Blockage — INSUFFICIENCY — Area of blocked arterioles

STROKE — Dead brain tissue

STROKE

Circle of Willis

Aneurysm

Basilar artery

Blood from a burst aneurysm

Circle of Willis

Basilar artery

Blocked artery

Blood clot

Brain in cross-section

Damage to the heart
- **Heart disease leading to heart attack:** Fat deposits and blockages form in the arteries that supply the heart with blood.
- **Congestive heart failure:** Heart becomes damaged and enlarged from working so hard to pump blood against the higher blood pressure.

Blocked artery

Damaged heart tissue

Enlarged heart

Normal heart

Narrowing of renal artery

Diseased kidney

Damage to the kidneys
- **Blood vessel damage:** Arteries become narrowed and stiff from high pressure. Blood flow to the kidneys is decreased. Receptors respond by recruiting mechanisms throughout the body to *raise* overall blood pressure even further.
- **Kidney disease leading to failure:** It becomes more and more difficult for the kidneys to remove impurities from the blood. Toxic materials accumulate.

Treatment of high blood pressure

The only way to detect high blood pressure early is to have your blood pressure measured by a healthcare professional. Secondary hypertension is treated by managing the disease that is causing it. Although primary hypertension cannot be cured, there are several ways to lower blood pressure and keep it controlled:

Diet and medication

Improvements in diet alone may be enough to control high blood pressure, especially in mild cases. Often, improvements in diet need to be combined with medication to control high blood pressure. Due to the vast number of mechanisms in the body that affect blood pressure, there are several different types of medications. Your physician will determine which is best for you and may eventually suggest taking more than one.

Diuretics decrease blood volume by causing more water and salt to be excreted in the urine.

Sympathetic nervous system blocking drugs cause the heart to slow down and beat less forcefully. They also decrease constriction of arteries throughout the body. *Examples are alpha, beta and adrenergic blockers.*

Vasodilators act directly on blood vessel walls or through other mechanisms to increase blood vessel diameter. *Examples are calcium channel blockers, ACE inhibitors, angiotensin II inhibitors, and angiotensin receptor blockers.*

Taking control of your blood pressure

- Maintain a low-fat diet.
- Decrease salt intake to less than a teaspoon per day (2000 mg).
- Shed extra weight to decrease strain on your heart.
- Don't smoke.
- Restrict caffeine and alcohol consumption.
- Follow all of your physician's instructions.
- Take prescribed medications as part of your daily routine.
- Consult your physician about an appropriate exercise plan and follow it.
- Measure blood pressure regularly at home.
- Continue taking medication even after your blood pressure has reached a good level.

Effective control of high blood pressure can prevent most of its complications.

Tissue — Arteriole — Nutrients — Capillaries — Venule — Waste — Capillaries

©Scientific Publishing Ltd., Elk Grove Village, IL USA
#1450

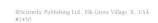
PLATE 8

Understanding Heart Disease

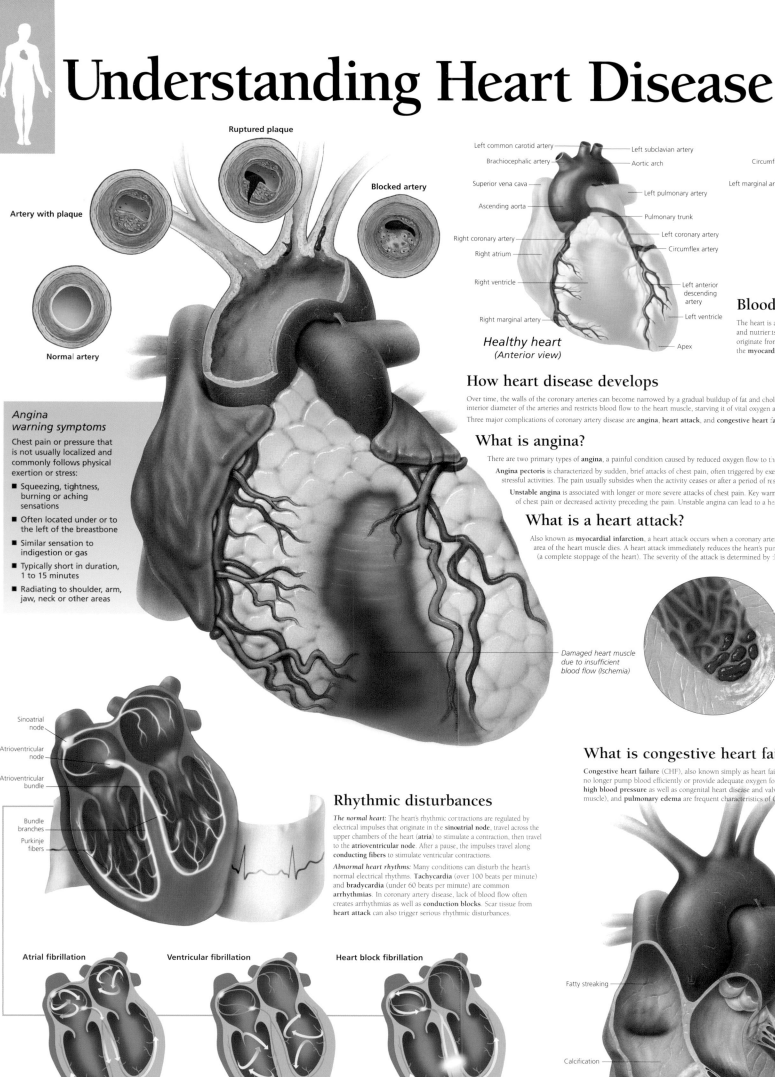

Ruptured plaque

Blocked artery

Artery with plaque

Normal artery

Healthy heart
(Anterior view)

Left common carotid artery — — Left subclavian artery
Brachiocephalic artery — — Aortic arch
Superior vena cava — — Left pulmonary artery
Ascending aorta — — Pulmonary trunk
Right coronary artery — — Left coronary artery
Right atrium — — Circumflex artery
Right ventricle — — Left anterior descending artery
Right marginal artery — — Left ventricle
— Apex

Healthy heart
(Posterior view)

Circumflex artery
Left marginal artery
Posterior descending artery

Blood supply and the heart

The heart is a powerful muscle that depends on a continuous flow of oxygen and nutrients. This blood supply is provided by **coronary arteries**, which originate from the aorta and branch out to deliver oxygenated blood throughout the **myocardium**, the muscular layer of the heart wall.

How heart disease develops

Over time, the walls of the coronary arteries can become narrowed by a gradual buildup of fat and cholesterol deposits called **plaque**. This process, **atherosclerosis**, reduces the interior diameter of the arteries and restricts blood flow to the heart muscle, starving it of vital oxygen and nutrients. The resulting condition is **coronary artery disease (CAD)**. Three major complications of coronary artery disease are **angina**, **heart attack**, and **congestive heart failure**.

What is angina?

There are two primary types of **angina**, a painful condition caused by reduced oxygen flow to the muscle fibers in the heart.

Angina pectoris is characterized by sudden, brief attacks of chest pain, often triggered by exercise and other strenuous or stressful activities. The pain usually subsides when the activity ceases or after a period of rest.

Unstable angina is associated with longer or more severe attacks of chest pain. Key warning signs are changing patterns of chest pain or decreased activity preceding the pain. Unstable angina can lead to a heart attack.

What is a heart attack?

Also known as **myocardial infarction**, a heart attack occurs when a coronary artery is suddenly blocked by a blood clot. Deprived of oxygen, the affected area of the heart muscle dies. A heart attack immediately reduces the heart's pumping ability and may lead to **cardiac arrythmias** and **cardiac arrest** (a complete stoppage of the heart). The severity of the attack is determined by the amount of heart muscle damage and the function of nearby arteries.

Damaged heart muscle due to insufficient blood flow (Ischemia)

Formation of blood clots in damaged heart muscle

What is congestive heart failure?

Congestive heart failure (CHF), also known simply as heart failure, is a condition in which the heart has become weak and can no longer pump blood efficiently or provide adequate oxygen for the brain and other organs. Causes of CHF include CAD and **high blood pressure** as well as congenital heart disease and valve disease. Enlarged heart, **hypertrophy** (thickening of the heart muscle), and **pulmonary edema** are frequent characteristics of CHF

Rhythmic disturbances

The normal heart: The heart's rhythmic contractions are regulated by electrical impulses that originate in the **sinoatrial node**, travel across the upper chambers of the heart (**atria**) to stimulate a contraction, then travel to the **atrioventricular node**. After a pause, the impulses travel along **conducting fibers** to stimulate ventricular contractions.

Abnormal heart rhythms: Many conditions can disturb the heart's normal electrical rhythms. **Tachycardia** (over 100 beats per minute) and **bradycardia** (under 60 beats per minute) are common **arrhythmias**. In coronary artery disease, lack of blood flow often creates arrhythmias as well as **conduction blocks**. Scar tissue from **heart attack** can also trigger serious rhythmic disturbances.

Sinoatrial node
Atrioventricular node
Atrioventricular bundle
Bundle branches
Purkinje fibers

Atrial fibrillation

Ventricular fibrillation

Heart block fibrillation

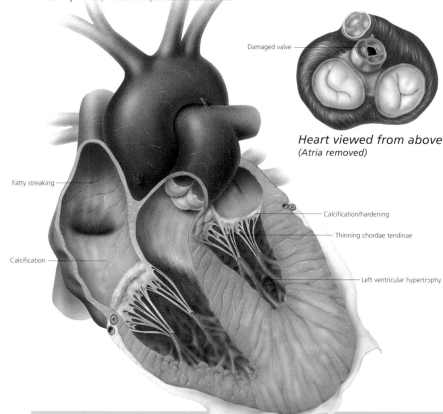

Heart viewed from above
(Atria removed)

Damaged valve
Calcification/hardening
Thinning chordae tendinae
Left ventricular hypertrophy
Fatty streaking
Calcification

Causes of coronary artery disease

The disease processes that lead to CAD have been attributed to many different causes. They include **genetic**, **age**, and **gender factors** as well as lifestyle or **modifiable risks**.

- High blood pressure
- Smoking
- High cholesterol
- Obesity
- Diabetes
- Inactive lifestyle
- Stress

A higher number of risk factors increases your chances of developing CAD.

Healthy lifestyle changes

By following recommended lifestyle changes, many risk factors for heart disease can be significantly reduced or controlled. Seeking treatment for **hypertension**, lowering **cholesterol** through diet and medication, quitting **smoking**, increasing **physical activity**, managing **diabetes**, and **losing weight** are all important steps to a healthier heart.

©Scientific Publishing Ltd., Elk Grove Village, IL, USA
#1454

PLATE 9

Understanding Stroke

What is stroke?

A **stroke** is a cerebral vascular accident that occurs when blood flow to the brain is suddenly interrupted by a **burst blood vessel** or a **blockage** in the brain's blood supply. Nerve cells in the affected part of the brain no longer receive oxygen and nutrients, and the result is temporary or permanent loss of function in the corresponding parts of the body.

Strokes are classified into two major categories:

- **Ischemic** stroke is the most common type, occurring in approximately 80 percent of all cases
- **Hemorrhagic** stroke is present in about 20 percent of stroke cases

What are the causes of stroke?

Every type of stroke has a specific physiological cause. In general, however, strokes are frequently caused by underlying medical conditions such as **high blood pressure**, **heart disease**, or **atherosclerosis** (narrowing of the arteries). Strokes may also be the result of **head injuries**, **aneurysms**, or **congenital defects** in the arteries of the brain.

ISCHEMIC

HEMORRHAGIC

Ischemic strokes happen when blood flow to the brain is blocked by clots or fragments that have become lodged within the blood vessels. The **origin of the clot** determines what type of ischemic stroke has occurred.

Embolic strokes are frequently caused by atrial fibrillation, a heart condition in which incomplete pumping of the heart's upper chambers results in the formation of clots.

Embolus

Cerebral embolism

A blood clot called an **embolus** forms in the circulatory system. Blockage occurs when the clot reaches vessels in the brain too small to let it pass.

Headaches and seizures can occur almost immediately.

Thrombus

Narrowed artery

There are three types of **hemorrhagic stroke**, which occurs when blood from a ruptured vessel accumulates and compresses surrounding brain tissue, injuring cells and interfering with brain function. The leaking vessel also interrupts **oxygen flow** to the brain. The amount of bleeding determines the severity of the stroke.

Normal   AVM

Treating high blood pressure, which strains the blood vessels and increases the risk of stroke, is one of the most important ways to help prevent risk of stroke.

Cerebral thrombosis

A blood clot or **thrombus** forms within an artery supplying blood to the brain. The most common type of stroke, thrombosis often results from damage to the arteries caused by fatty deposit buildups (atherosclerosis).

Symptoms such as loss of feeling, speech problems and seizures may occur gradually, over a period of minutes or hours.

Circle of Willis

Burst aneurysm

Basilar artery

Subarachnoid

A ruptured blood vessel on the surface of the brain bleeds into the space **between the skull and the brain**.

As the vessel weakens, warning signs such as sudden headaches and light-sensitivity may be present for days or weeks.

Area of burst arterioles

Arteriovenous malformation (AVM)

A rupture occurs within a cluster of abnormally formed blood vessels in the brain.

Symptoms may include migraine-like headache, numbness, muscle weakness and seizures.

Intracerebral

Blood from a **ruptured artery in the brain** is released into surrounding brain tissue.

The symptoms usually occur suddenly and can include headache, nausea and marked changes in mental state.

Cerebrovascular insufficiency:

A series of mini-strokes occurs in the smaller vessels of the brain. Tiny arterioles bulge, then burst from high pressure or become blocked by small blood clots.

There are no symptoms until damage accumulates over time.

Brain in cross-section

Stroke risk factors

- High blood pressure
- High blood cholesterol
- Atherosclerosis
- Heart disease/heart abnormalities
- Adult-onset diabetes
- Family history of stroke
- Previous TIA
- Cigarette smoking
- Excess weight
- Heavy alcohol consumption
- Inactive lifestyle

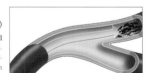

Transient ischemic attack (TIA)

A temporary blockage of blood flow to the brain is caused by **small emboli** that break up and dissolve shortly after lodging in vessel walls. Mild stroke-like symptoms can last for minutes or up to 24 hours.

Symptoms lasting over 24 hours are considered a stroke. TIAs are often warning signs of future ischemic stroke and should be treated immediately.

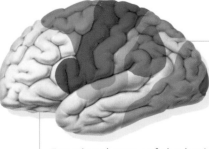
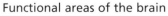

Functional areas of the brain

- Primary motor area
- Secondary motor area
- Primary somatosensory area
- Secondary somatosensory area
- Primary visual area
- Secondary visual area
- Primary acoustic area
- Secondary acoustic area
- Sensory speech area

Effects of strokes

Three factors influence the effects of a stroke:
- What type of stroke was it?
- Where did the stroke occur?
- How much injury was caused?

The location of the stroke is especially critical in understanding which parts of the body will be most affected. A stroke near the back of the brain will often cause changes in vision. A stroke on the right side of the brain will affect neurological function on the left (opposing) side of the body.

Right brain strokes may cause:
- Paralysis of the left arm, leg and side of face
- Less or impairment of analytical skills
- Problems with spatial perception
- Sudden, impulsive behavior
- Short-term memory loss

Left brain strokes may cause:
- Paralysis of the right arm, leg and side of face
- Difficulty speaking or understanding language (aphasia)
- Slow and cautious behavior
- Difficulty with conceptual thinking
- Memory loss and difficulty learning new tasks

Stroke symptoms

Most strokes share these warning signs and symptoms:
- Sudden or severe headache
- Dizziness or loss of balance
- Double vision or blurring in one or both eyes
- Difficulty in swallowing
- Weakness or numbness on one side of the body
- Difficulty in speaking or understanding others
- Confusion or difficulty thinking
- Sudden loss of bowel or bladder control

Call 911 immediately for help if you or someone you know experiences any of these symptoms of stroke.

Stroke rehabilitation

The time it takes to recover from a stroke and the amount of recovery possible depend on the amount of damage that occurred to the brain.

Regardless of the type of stroke, early intervention and treatment—within a few hours of the onset of the stroke–are critical in possibly preventing further brain injury and promoting long-term recovery.

- Diagnostic tests such as CT scans and MRI are used to determine the nature and extent of the stroke.
- Stroke rehabilitation can include physical, speech and occupational therapies.
- Recovery usually begins within the first few weeks and speech and function may continue to improve gradually for a year or more after the stroke.

PLATE 10

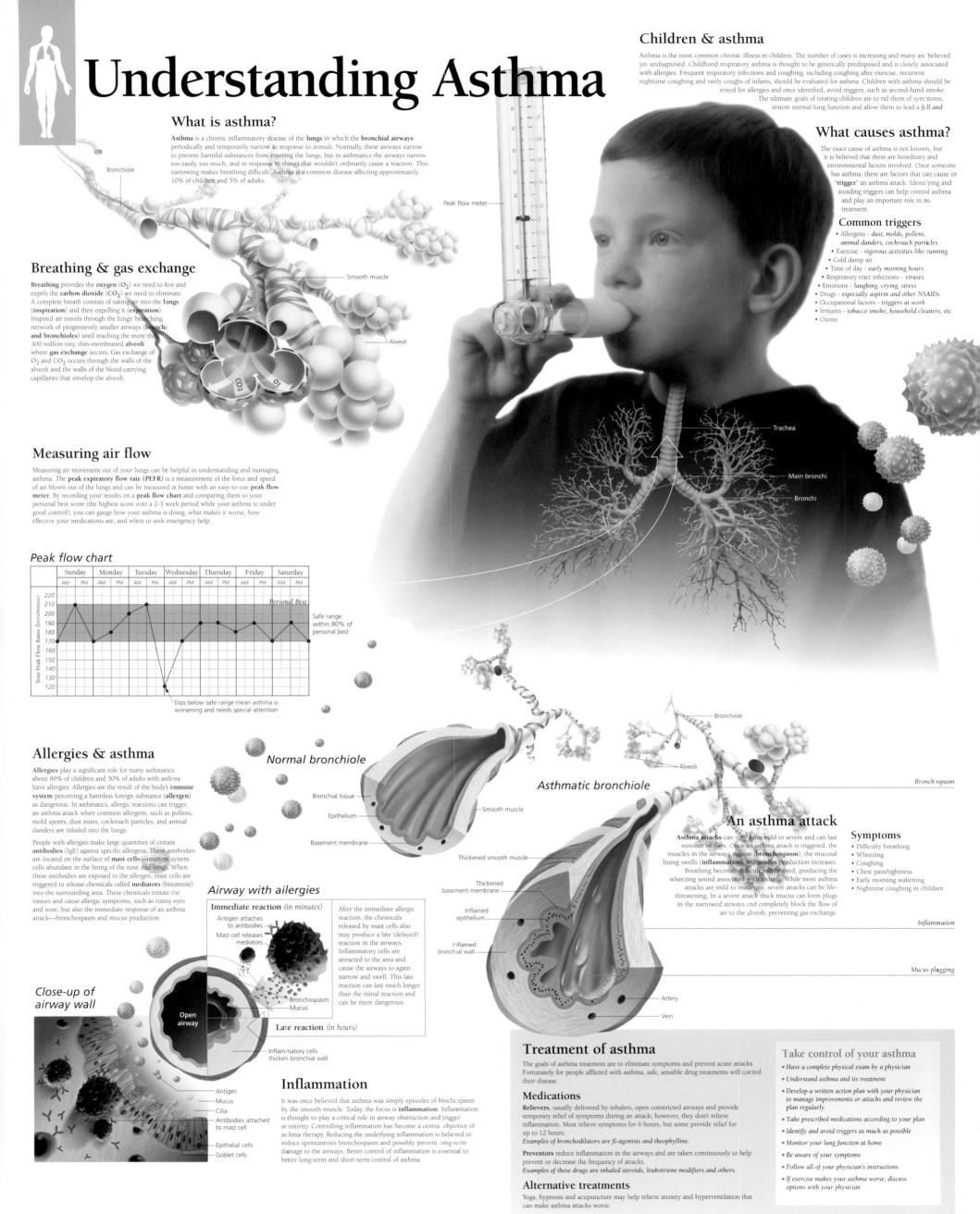

Understanding Asthma

What is asthma?

Asthma is a chronic inflammatory disease of the lungs in which the **bronchial airways** periodically and temporarily narrow in response to stimuli. Normally, these airways narrow to prevent harmful substances from entering the lungs, but in asthmatics the airways narrow too easily, too much, and in response to things that wouldn't ordinarily cause a reaction. This narrowing makes breathing difficult. Asthma is a common disease affecting approximately 10% of children and 5% of adults.

Breathing & gas exchange

Breathing provides the **oxygen (O$_2$)** we need to live and expels the **carbon dioxide (CO$_2$)** we need to eliminate. A complete breath consists of taking air into the **lungs** (**inspiration**) and then expelling it (**expiration**). Inspired air travels through the lungs' branching network of progressively smaller airways (**bronchi and bronchioles**) until reaching the more than 300 million tiny, thin-membraned **alveoli** where **gas exchange** occurs. Gas exchange of O$_2$ and CO$_2$ occurs through the walls of the alveoli and the walls of the blood-carrying capillaries that envelop the alveoli.

Measuring air flow

Measuring air movement out of your lungs can be helpful in understanding and managing asthma. The **peak expiratory flow rate (PEFR)** is a measurement of the force and speed of air blown out of the lungs and can be measured at home with an easy-to-use **peak flow meter**. By recording your results on a **peak flow chart** and comparing them to your personal best score (the highest score over a 2-3 week period while your asthma is under good control), you can gauge how your asthma is doing, what makes it worse, how effective your medications are, and when to seek emergency help.

Peak flow chart

	Sunday		Monday		Tuesday		Wednesday		Thursday		Friday		Saturday	
	AM	PM	AM	PM	AM	PM	AM	PM	AM	PM	AM	PM	AM	PM

Personal Best

Safe range within 80% of personal best

Your Peak Flow Flow Rates (liters/minute): 220 210 200 190 180 170 160 150 140 130 120

Dips below safe range mean asthma is worsening and needs special attention

Allergies & asthma

Allergies play a significant role for many asthmatics: about 80% of children and 50% of adults with asthma have allergies. Allergies are the result of the body's **immune system** perceiving a harmless foreign substance (**allergen**) as dangerous. In asthmatics, allergic reactions can trigger an asthma attack when common allergens, such as pollens, mold spores, dust mites, cockroach particles, and animal danders are inhaled into the lungs.

People with allergies make large quantities of certain **antibodies** (IgE) against specific allergens. These antibodies are located on the surface of **mast cells**—immune system cells abundant in the lining of the nose and lungs. When these antibodies are exposed to the allergen, mast cells are triggered to release chemicals called **mediators** (histamine) into the surrounding area. These chemicals irritate the tissues and cause allergic symptoms, such as runny eyes and nose, but also the immediate response of an asthma attack—bronchospasm and mucus production.

Close-up of airway wall

Open airway

Antigen
Mucus
Cilia
Antibodies attached to mast cell
Epithelial cells
Goblet cells

Children & asthma

Asthma is the most common chronic illness in children. The number of cases is increasing and many are believed yet undiagnosed. Childhood respiratory asthma is thought to be genetically predisposed and is closely associated with allergies. Frequent respiratory infections and coughing, including coughing after exercise, recurrent nighttime coughing and rattly coughs of infants, should be evaluated for asthma. Children with asthma should be tested for allergies and once identified, avoid triggers, such as second-hand smoke. The ultimate goals of treating children are to rid them of symptoms, restore normal lung function and allow them to lead a *full and*

Peak flow meter

Smooth muscle
Alveoli
Bronchiole

Trachea
Main bronchi
Bronchi

What causes asthma?

The exact cause of asthma is not known, but it is believed that there are hereditary and environmental factors involved. Once someone has asthma, there are factors that can cause or "**trigger**" an asthma attack. Identifying and avoiding triggers can help control asthma and play an important role in its treatment.

Common triggers

- Allergens - *dust, molds, pollens, animal danders, cockroach particles*
- Exercise - *vigorous activities like running*
- Cold damp air
- Time of day - *early morning hours*
- Respiratory tract infections - *viruses*
- Emotions - *laughing, crying, stress*
- Drugs - *especially aspirin and other NSAIDs*
- Occupational factors - *triggers at work*
- Irritants - *tobacco smoke, household cleaners, etc.*
- Ozone

Normal bronchiole

Bronchial tissue
Epithelium
Basement membrane
Smooth muscle

Asthmatic bronchiole

Thickened smooth muscle
Thickened basement membrane
Inflamed epithelium
Inflamed bronchial wall
Artery
Vein

Bronchiole
Alveoli

Bronchospasm
Inflammation
Mucus plugging

Airway with allergies

Immediate reaction (*in minutes*)

Antigen attaches to antibodies
Mast cell releases mediators

After the immediate allergic reaction, the chemicals released by mast cells also may produce a late (delayed) reaction in the airways. Inflammatory cells are attracted to the area and cause the airways to again narrow and swell. This late reaction can last much longer than the initial reaction and can be more dangerous.

Bronchospasm
Mucus

Late reaction (*in hours*)

Inflammatory cells thicken bronchial wall

An asthma attack

Asthma attacks can vary from mild to severe and can last minutes or days. Once an asthma attack is triggered, the muscles in the airways tighten (**bronchospasm**), the mucosal lining swells (**inflammation**) and mucus production increases. Breathing becomes difficult and labored, producing the wheezing sound associated with asthma. While most asthma attacks are mild to moderate, severe attacks can be life-threatening. In a severe attack thick mucus can form plugs in the narrowed airways and completely block the flow of air to the alveoli, preventing gas exchange.

Symptoms

- Difficulty breathing
- Wheezing
- Coughing
- Chest pain/tightness
- Early morning wakening
- Nighttime coughing in children

Inflammation

It was once believed that asthma was simply episodes of bronchospasm by the smooth muscle. Today, the focus is **inflammation**. Inflammation is thought to play a critical role in airway obstruction and trigger sensitivity. Controlling inflammation has become a central objective of asthma therapy. Reducing the underlying inflammation is believed to reduce spontaneous bronchospasm and possibly prevent long-term damage to the airways. Better control of inflammation is essential to better long-term and short-term control of asthma.

Treatment of asthma

The goals of asthma treatment are to eliminate symptoms and prevent acute attacks. Fortunately for people afflicted with asthma, safe, sensible drug treatments will control their disease.

Medications

Relievers, usually delivered by inhalers, open constricted airways and provide temporary relief of symptoms during an attack; however, they don't relieve inflammation. Most relieve symptoms for 6 hours, but some provide relief for up to 12 hours.
Examples of bronchodilators are ß-agonists and theophylline.

Preventors reduce inflammation in the airways and are taken continuously to help prevent or decrease the frequency of attacks.
Examples of these drugs are inhaled steroids, leukotriene modifiers and others.

Alternative treatments

Yoga, hypnosis and acupuncture may help relieve anxiety and hyperventilation that can make asthma attacks worse.

Take control of your asthma

- *Have a complete physical exam by a physician*
- *Understand asthma and its treatment*
- *Develop a written action plan with your physician to manage improvements or attacks and review the plan regularly*
- *Take prescribed medications according to your plan*
- *Identify and avoid triggers as much as possible*
- *Monitor your lung function at home*
- *Be aware of your symptoms*
- *Follow all of your physician's instructions*
- *If exercise makes your asthma worse, discuss options with your physician*

PLATE 11

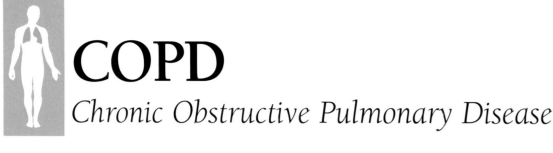

COPD
Chronic Obstructive Pulmonary Disease

Chronic Obstructive Pulmonary Disease (COPD)

Chronic Obstructive Pulmonary Disease (COPD), also called chronic obstructive lung disease, is a name used for two related diseases of the respiratory system: **emphysema** and **chronic bronchitis**. In many individuals these diseases occur together, although there may be more symptoms of one than the other. The majority of individuals with COPD have a long history of cigarette smoking.

COPD gradually worsens with time. Initially there may be only a mild shortness of breath and occasional coughing. A chronic cough then develops with a clear, colorless sputum. As the disease progresses, the cough worsens and more effort is needed to get air into and out of the lungs. In later stages, the heart might become affected. Eventually death occurs when the functioning of the lungs and heart is no longer adequate to supply oxygen to the body's organs and tissues.

Approximately 80%-90% of COPD cases are caused by smoking. Air pollution and occupational exposures play a role, especially when combined with cigarette smoking. By the time symptoms of COPD appear—typically cough, shortness of breath and difficulty tolerating exercise—damage has already occurred to your lungs.

Emphysema

Signs & symptoms:
• Shortness of breath
• Chronic, mild cough that may produce sputum
• Weight loss

On average, the lungs contain 300 million elastic air sacs, called alveoli, in which oxygen is added to the blood and carbon dioxide is removed from it. Emphysema occurs when there is permanent damage to the alveoli and they lose their natural elasticity, become over stretched and rupture, preventing the lungs from properly functioning. This results in the bloodstream not receiving the required amounts of oxygen.

What causes emphysema?
The normal lung has a unique balance between two chemicals with opposing actions. The elastic fibers allow the lung to expand and contract. When the chemical balance is altered the lungs lose the ability to protect themselves against the destruction of these elastic fibers. Smoking is responsible for the majority (80%-90%) of emphysema cases. Individuals born with a protein deficiency known as alpha-1 antitrypsin (AAT) may develop to an inherited form of emphysema.

Chronic bronchitis

Signs & symptoms:
• Chronic cough that produces mucus
• Shortness of breath

This disorder consists of chronic inflammation and thickening of the lining of the bronchial tubes. Pushing the air through narrowed airways becomes harder and harder. In addition, the inflammation causes the glands of the bronchial tubes to produce excessive amounts of mucus, increasing congestion in the lungs and further inhibiting the ability to breathe. Air flow is hindered and the lungs are endangered.

The primary symptom of chronic bronchitis (as distinct from emphysema) is a chronic cough that produces a large amount of mucus and has persisted for at least 3 months of the year for more than 2 consecutive years. Once the bronchial tubes have been irritated over a long period of time, excessive mucus is produced constantly.

What causes chronic bronchitis?
In addition to smoking, higher rates of chronic bronchitis are found among coal miners, grain handlers, metal molders and other workers exposed to dust.

Breathing

All humans need **oxygen** to burn nutrients, which release the energy we need to live. Through breathing, our respiratory system provides this needed oxygen and expels the **carbon dioxide** we need to eliminate. A complete breath includes taking air into the lungs (**inspiration**) and then expelling it (**expiration**). A normal adult inhales about 16 pints of air per minute while awake and about 6 to 8 pints per minute while asleep. During exercise or under stressful situations, the body's demand for oxygen increases and the rate of breathing increases.

Enlargement of lung tissue:
(*left*) From a normal lung.
(*right*) From a lung with emphysema. In emphysema, lung tissue is destroyed, resulting in fewer and larger alveoli

Labels: Frontal sinus, Superior nasal concha, Sphenoid sinus, Middle nasal concha, Inferior nasal concha, Nasopharynx, Soft palate, Oropharynx, Epiglottis, Thyroid cartilage, Esophagus, Cricoid cartilage, Trachea

Normal alveoli, Damaged alveoli, Alveolar sac, Capillaries, Alveolus, O2, CO2

Bronchospasm, Mucus, Open airway, Thickened bronchial wall

Thickened smooth muscle, Thickened basement membrane, Inflamed epithelium, Inflamed bronchial wall, Mucus, Vein, Artery

Taking control of your COPD

▪ Don't smoke.
▪ Avoid exposures to dusts and fumes.
▪ Avoid air pollution and cigarette smoke.
  ▪ Limit activities during air pollution and ozone alerts.
    ▪ Avoid excessive heat, cold and very high altitudes. (Most COPD patients can travel on commercial airlines with pressurized cabins.)
    ▪ Limit exposure to people with respiratory infections, colds and the flu.
    ▪ Maintain a normal weight. Being over- or underweight can worsen the conditions of COPD.
  ▪ Drink lots of fluids to loosen sputum so it can be easily coughed up.
▪ Follow a nutritious, well-balanced diet.
▪ Follow all of your physician's instructions.
▪ Take prescribed medications as part of your daily routine.
▪ Don't take other people's medications.
▪ Consult your physician about an appropriate exercise plan and follow it.

Effective control of COPD can prevent most of its complications.

How is Chronic Obstructive Pulmonary Disease detected?

There are no accurate methods to predict an individual's chance of developing COPD. None of the current ways to diagnose COPD detects the disease before irreversible lung damage occurs.

Pulmonary function tests
Pulmonary function tests (PFTs) are used to determine lung characteristics and capabilities. These tests include:
• **Total lung capacity:** the amount of air the lungs can hold.
• **Forced expiratory volume:** how quickly air moves in and out of the lungs.
• **Arterial blood gas - pulse oximetry:** how efficiently the lungs transfer oxygen from the air into the blood.
• **Arterial blood gas:** how efficiently the lungs remove carbon dioxide from the blood.
• **X-ray:** in moderate to severe cases, a reasonably accurate diagnosis of COPD can be made with a plain chest x-ray and CAT (computerized axial tomography) scanning.

In most cases, it is necessary to compare the results of several tests in order to make the correct diagnosis, and to repeat some tests at intervals to determine the rate of disease progression or improvement. Test results are compared to values considered healthy for an individual's sex, age, weight, height and race.

How is Chronic Obstructive Pulmonary Disease treated?

Although there is no cure for COPD, the disease can be prevented in many cases. In almost all cases the symptoms can be reduced. Survival of individuals with COPD is closely related to the level of their lung function when they are diagnosed and the rate at which they lose this function. The median survival is about 10 years for those with COPD who have lost approximately two-thirds of their normally expected lung function at diagnosis.

There are a number of treatments which can help individuals with COPD. These treatments can be separated into several categories:
I.   **Bronchodilators** help open narrowed bronchus and bronchial tubes.
II. **Anti-inflammatories (steroids)** reduce inflammation of the airway walls.
III. **Continuous oxygen therapy** is recommended for individuals with low blood oxygen levels.
IV. **Lung reduction surgery** removes damaged areas of the lung so it can perform more efficiently.
V.   **Transplant surgery** is a highly complex procedure that is considered a viable option only in a select group of individuals.
VI. **Pulmonary rehabilitation programs** can be combined with medical treatment to improve overall physical endurance and sense of well-being.

Medication and exercise

Medications for COPD can be given in several forms. The two most common are inhaled or pill medications. Metered-dose inhalers (MDIs) are a convenient, safe way to deliver medication. Because the medication goes directly to the lungs, smaller doses can be used with minimal side effects. Proper technique in using hand-held inhalers is very important to their effectiveness.

Frequently prescribed medications for COPD patients include:
Bronchodilators to open narrowed airways
Corticosteroids or steroids to reduce inflammation
Antibiotics to fight respiratory infections
Expectorants to loosen and expel mucus secretions from airways
Diuretics to help excrete excess body fluids
Digitalis to strengthen the force of the heartbeat
Other drugs may include tranquilizers, pain killers and cough suppressants.

After smoking cessation, exercise is important to the nonmedical treatment of COPD. Exercise builds and maintains strength, maintains flexibility of the bones and joints and builds stamina to increase the amount of activity possible for a COPD patient. A physician, respiratory therapist or physical therapist should always be consulted before setting up a specific exercise program.

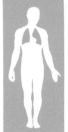

The Effects of Smoking

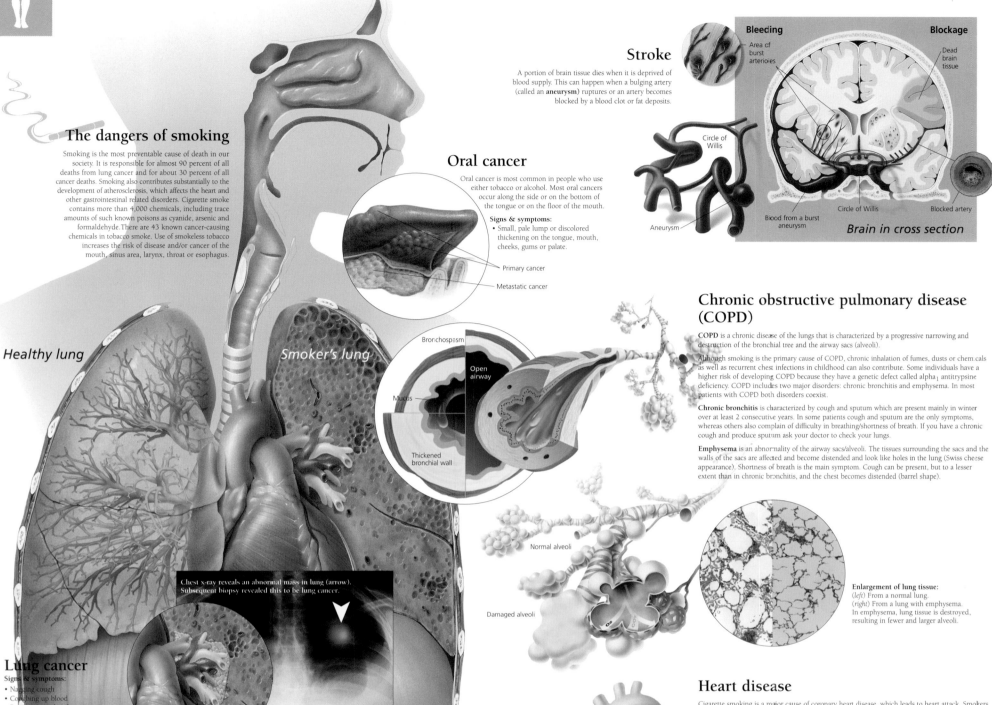

The dangers of smoking

Smoking is the most preventable cause of death in our society. It is responsible for almost 90 percent of all deaths from lung cancer and for about 30 percent of all cancer deaths. Smoking also contributes substantially to the development of atherosclerosis, which affects the heart and other gastrointestinal related disorders. Cigarette smoke contains more than 4,000 chemicals, including trace amounts of such known poisons as cyanide, arsenic and formaldehyde. There are 43 known cancer-causing chemicals in tobacco smoke. Use of smokeless tobacco increases the risk of disease and/or cancer of the mouth, sinus area, larynx, throat or esophagus.

Healthy lung

Smoker's lung

Chest x-ray reveals an abnormal mass in lung (arrow). Subsequent biopsy revealed this to be lung cancer.

Lung cancer
Signs & symptoms:
• Nagging cough
• Coughing up blood
• Persistent attacks of pneumonia, bronchitis or chest pain

Approximately 85 percent of the cases of lung cancer that occur each year can be traced to smoking. A person who smokes 2 packs of cigarettes or more daily for 20 years has a 60 to 70 fold increased risk of cancer compared to a nonsmoker. The risk of lung cancer increases with the number of cigarettes that are smoked each day, the number of years smoked, the amount of smoke that is inhaled and the amount of tar and nicotine in the cigarettes that are smoked.

Cancer of the esophagus
Signs & symptoms:
• Difficulty in swallowing
• Chest pain or discomfort
• Weight loss

Tobacco use can cause esophageal cancer by damaging the structure of cells that line the inside of the esophagus. The longer a person uses tobacco the higher the risk.

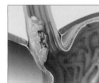

Gastric ulcers
Signs & symptoms:
• Gnawing or burning pain in the abdomen
• Nausea, vomiting
• Loss of appetite and weight

The effects of prolonged exposure to smoking contribute to a buildup of stomach acids that erode the protective lining of the stomach. Gnawing or burning pain in the abdomen between the breastbone and the navel is the most common symptom, often occurring between meals and in the early hours of the morning. The pain can last for anything from a few minutes to a few hours and may be relieved by eating or by taking antacids. Smoking slows the healing of existing ulcers and also contributes to ulcer recurrence.

Stomach cancer
Stomach cancer does not usually produce symptoms in the early stages of its development. It is known that stomach cancer can develop from the symptoms of gastric ulcers, and that excessive smoking increases a person's risk of developing the disease.

Other GI diseases
Smoking has also been indicated as a risk factor for Crohn's disease and possibly gallstones.

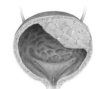

Bladder cancer
Signs & symptoms:
• Blood in the urine
• Pelvic pain
• Difficulty in voiding urine

Bladder cancer is prevalent among smokers over 40. Men are 4 times more likely than women to get bladder cancer. The presence of blood in the urine without pain or discomfort is the most common early symptom.

Oral cancer
Oral cancer is most common in people who use either tobacco or alcohol. Most oral cancers occur along the side or on the bottom of the tongue or on the floor of the mouth.

Signs & symptoms:
• Small, pale lump or discolored thickening on the tongue, mouth, cheeks, gums or palate.

Primary cancer

Metastatic cancer

Bronchospasm

Open airway

Mucus

Thickened bronchial wall

Stroke
A portion of brain tissue dies when it is deprived of blood supply. This can happen when a bulging artery (called an **aneurysm**) ruptures or an artery becomes blocked by a blood clot or fat deposits.

Bleeding

Blockage

Area of burst arteries

Dead brain tissue

Circle of Willis

Aneurysm

Blood from a burst aneurysm

Circle of Willis

Blocked artery

Brain in cross section

Chronic obstructive pulmonary disease (COPD)

COPD is a chronic disease of the lungs that is characterized by a progressive narrowing and destruction of the bronchial tree and the airway sacs (alveoli).

Although smoking is the primary cause of COPD, chronic inhalation of fumes, dusts or chemicals as well as recurrent chest infections in childhood can also contribute. Some individuals have a higher risk of developing COPD because they have a genetic defect called alpha$_1$ antitrypsine deficiency. COPD includes two major disorders: chronic bronchitis and emphysema. In most patients with COPD both disorders coexist.

Chronic bronchitis is characterized by cough and sputum which are present mainly in winter over at least 2 consecutive years. In some patients cough and sputum are the only symptoms, whereas others also complain of difficulty in breathing/shortness of breath. If you have a chronic cough and produce sputum ask your doctor to check your lungs.

Emphysema is an abnormality of the airway sacs/alveoli. The tissues surrounding the sacs and the walls of the sacs are affected and become distended and look like holes in the lung (Swiss cheese appearance). Shortness of breath is the main symptom. Cough can be present, but to a lesser extent than in chronic bronchitis, and the chest becomes distended (barrel shape).

Normal alveoli

Damaged alveoli

Enlargement of lung tissue:
(*left*) From a normal lung.
(*right*) From a lung with emphysema.
In emphysema, lung tissue is destroyed, resulting in fewer and larger alveoli.

Heart disease

Cigarette smoking is a major cause of coronary heart disease, which leads to heart attack. Smokers have a greater risk of developing chronic disorders such as **atherosclerosis** (clogged arteries) and other damaging effects to the cardiovascular system. Smoking increases the risk of coronary heart disease by itself, and by acting with other risk factors to greatly increase risk. The nicotine and carbon monoxide in cigarette smoke prevent the effective release of oxygen into the bloodstream, damaging the cardiovascular system in many ways.

Blocked coronary artery

Damage to the heart
Heart disease leading to heart attack:
Fat deposits and blockages form in the arteries that supply the heart with blood.
Congestive heart failure:
Heart becomes damaged and enlarged from working so hard to pump blood against the higher blood pressure.

Enlarged heart

Normal heart

Damaged heart tissue

Women's health issues:
Risk factors and pregnancy

Using tobacco increases a woman's risk of chronic health problems including pulmonary complications and premature death. Studies suggest that cigarette smoking dramatically increases the risk of heart disease among premenopausal women who are also taking birth control pills. Studies show that mothers who smoke a pack or more of cigarettes a day consistently produce smaller babies than do non-smokers. The carbon monoxide inhaled with cigarette smoke reaches the fetus and diminishes its ability to absorb oxygen, resulting in significant oxygen deprivation. Other complications include decreased blood flow, which diminishes the transfer of essential nutrients from mother to fetus. A small baby is generally weaker and more vulnerable to illness than one of average size. Smokers are more apt to have their pregnancy end in premature birth, miscarriage or stillbirth. Research also suggests that infants are more likely to die from **Sudden Infant Death Syndrome (SIDS)** if their mothers smoke during and after pregnancy.

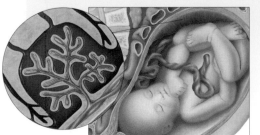

Enlargement of placental tissue:
Nicotine stimulates the release of hormones that constrict the vessels supplying blood to the placenta and uterus, diminishing the transfer of essential nutrients from mother to fetus.

Cancers
Smoking exposes the body to many cancer-causing chemicals that flow through the body. Tobacco byproducts have been found in the cervical mucus in women who smoke. Researchers believe these substances damage the structure of the cells in the cervix and may contribute to the development of cancers.

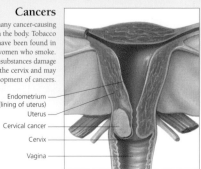

Endometrium (lining of uterus)

Uterus

Cervical cancer

Cervix

Vagina

PLATE 13

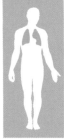

The Common Cold vs. the Flu

What is a common cold?

The common cold is an infection of the nose and throat caused by a virus (a microscopic infectious agent or 'germ'). Colds can involve the **sinuses**, **ears**, **bronchial tubes** and the **eustachian tube**, which connects the middle ear and throat, windpipe, voice box and airways. Infection with a cold virus is less severe than influenza, but mild cases of flu can sometimes appear similar to a common cold. Cold symptoms include sneezing, runny or blocked nose, sore throat, cough and low grade fever. Most common colds occur gradually and last two to three days; severe colds can last up to two weeks.

How a cold virus infection occurs

The cold virus is present in the mucus and saliva of an infected person. You can catch a cold when the cold virus enters your nasal passages. This may be through **contaminated fingers** or **airborne droplets from coughs and sneezes**. The virus enters healthy cells in the nose and the adenoid, which become infected and produce new virus particles. As cells die, new cold viruses are released and infect other cells. Only small doses of the virus (2-30) particles are necessary to produce an infection. At present, over 200 cold viruses have been identified.

Treating a cold

There are no medications currently available that can cure the common cold, but symptoms can be treated or alleviated with nonprescription **analgesics** such as paracetamol and ibuprofen, as well as over-the-counter **decongestants**, **cough syrups** and **throat lozenges**. (Check with your physician prior to taking any medication if you are already taking prescription or over-the-counter drugs.) Plenty of rest and fluids to thin mucus secretions are also important.

Aspirin and colds/flu

Aspirin should never be given to children or teenagers who have cold or flu-like symptoms, particularly fever, due to the risk of a rare but dangerous complication of influenza known as **Reyes syndrome**.

Inflammation of bronchial airway

- Bronchospasm
- Mucus
- Open airway
- Thickened bronchial wall

What is the flu?

"Flu" is the common name for **influenza**, a viral illness of the **respiratory tract**. Infection occurs in the **nose**, **throat**, **bronchial tubes** and **lungs**. Symptoms, such as **muscle aches**, **fever** and **chills**, usually begin suddenly, are more severe and last longer than common cold symptoms. Because infection with an influenza virus can damage the lungs, it can lead to significant complications such as **pneumonia**. Those most at risk of serious complications of influenza are children, older people (over 65), people with chronic illnesses (such as asthma, heart disease or diabetes) and people with compromised immune systems.

How flu virus is transmitted

The coughing, sneezing and **talking** of an infected person releases millions of tiny droplets containing the virus into the air. Once inhaled, they enter the body and reproduce in healthy cells, infecting the lining of the respiratory tract. Influenza virus is **highly contagious** and can be transmitted up to seven days after symptoms begin.

Respiratory mucosa

- Serous cell
- Mucous cell
- Tubule
- Lamina propria
- Goblet cell
- Pseudostratified columnar epithelium
- Mucus
- Cilia
- Mucous gland

Inflamed respiratory mucosa

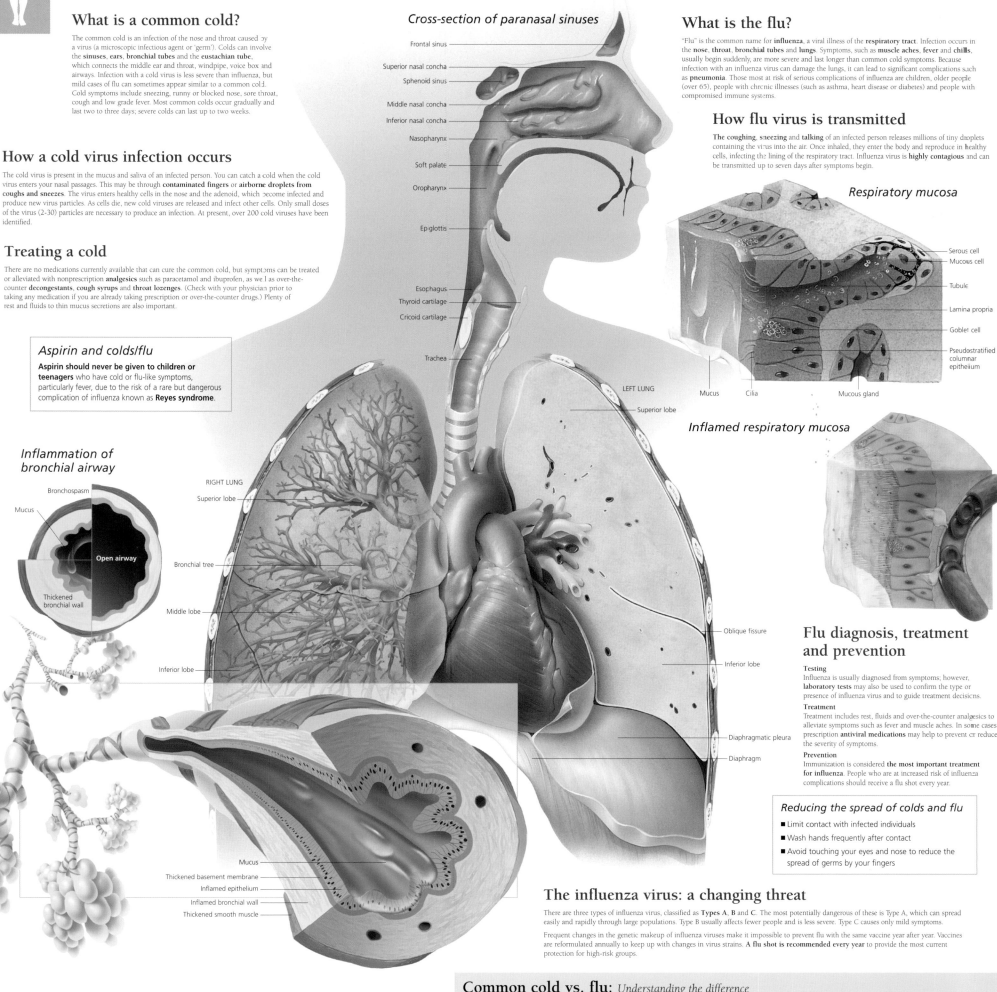

Cross-section of paranasal sinuses

- Frontal sinus
- Superior nasal concha
- Sphenoid sinus
- Middle nasal concha
- Inferior nasal concha
- Nasopharynx
- Soft palate
- Oropharynx
- Epiglottis
- Esophagus
- Thyroid cartilage
- Cricoid cartilage
- Trachea

- LEFT LUNG
- Superior lobe

- RIGHT LUNG
- Superior lobe
- Bronchial tree
- Middle lobe
- Inferior lobe

- Oblique fissure
- Inferior lobe
- Diaphragmatic pleura
- Diaphragm

- Mucus
- Thickened basement membrane
- Inflamed epithelium
- Inflamed bronchial wall
- Thickened smooth muscle

Flu diagnosis, treatment and prevention

Testing
Influenza is usually diagnosed from symptoms; however, **laboratory tests** may also be used to confirm the type or presence of influenza virus and to guide treatment decisions.

Treatment
Treatment includes rest, fluids and over-the-counter analgesics to alleviate symptoms such as fever and muscle aches. In some cases prescription **antiviral medications** may help to prevent or reduce the severity of symptoms.

Prevention
Immunization is considered **the most important treatment for influenza**. People who are at increased risk of influenza complications should receive a flu shot every year.

Reducing the spread of colds and flu

- Limit contact with infected individuals
- Wash hands frequently after contact
- Avoid touching your eyes and nose to reduce the spread of germs by your fingers

The influenza virus: a changing threat

There are three types of influenza virus, classified as **Types A**, **B** and **C**. The most potentially dangerous of these is Type A, which can spread easily and rapidly through large populations. Type B usually affects fewer people and is less severe. Type C causes only mild symptoms.

Frequent changes in the genetic makeup of influenza viruses make it impossible to prevent flu with the same vaccine year after year. Vaccines are reformulated annually to keep up with changes in virus strains. **A flu shot is recommended every year** to provide the most current protection for high-risk groups.

Middle ear infections

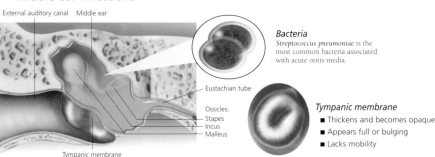

- External auditory canal
- Middle ear
- Eustachian tube
- Ossicles:
  - Stapes
  - Incus
  - Malleus
- Tympanic membrane

Bacteria
Streptococcus pneumoniae is the most common bacteria associated with acute otitis media.

Tympanic membrane
- Thickens and becomes opaque
- Appears full or bulging
- Lacks mobility

Common cold vs. flu: *Understanding the difference*

COMMON COLD	INFLUENZA
Primary symptoms – gradual onset	**Primary symptoms – acute onset**
Runny nose, sneezing, watery eyes	Severe headache and/or muscle aches
Sore or scratchy throat	Fever of 39-40°C or 102-104°F (may last 3-4 days)
Mild cough	Fatigue/exhaustion (may last two weeks or more)
Fatigue	Chills
Occasional low grade fever (<38.5°C or 101°F)	Cough (can become severe)
Complications	**Complications**
Middle ear infections (otitis media)	Pneumonia
Acute bacterial sinusitis	Bronchial, ear and sinus infections
Asthma attacks and worsening of chronic bronchitis	Worsening of chronic conditions such as asthma, congestive heart failure and diabetes
Prevention	**Prevention**
No preventive treatment	Annual flu shots recommended for high-risk groups
	Sometimes antiviral medications may be used to prevent flu and reduce symptom duration and severity

PLATE 14

Understanding Sinusitis

What is sinusitis?

Sinusitis is an inflammation of the lining of the **paranasal sinuses**, hollow cavities within the bones of the face behind the eyes and around the nose. There are four pairs of sinuses: frontal, maxillary, ethmoid and sphenoid. They are joined by a continuous mucous membrane that produces **mucus**, a slippery secretion that moistens the nasal passages and traps dirt particles from incoming air. Tiny hairs in the membrane (**cilia**) move the mucus and particles into the nasal cavity through very small openings in the sinuses called **ostia**. If the mucous membranes become inflamed by colds or allergies, swelling can block normal drainage through these openings, leading to sinus inflammation and infection.

Sinus pain

When the sinuses are blocked, air, pus and other secretions can become trapped and put pressure on the sinus walls, causing significant pain. Swollen membranes can also prevent air from entering a sinus cavity, creating a painful vacuum.

Sinusitis vs. Rhinitis

Although many of the symptoms of sinusitis and the common cold (rhinitis) can appear similar, **sinusitis** refers specifically to inflammation of mucous membranes within the sinuses. In rhinitis, inflammation is present in the membranes of the nasal cavity. However, sinusitis frequently occurs in conjunction with rhinitis.

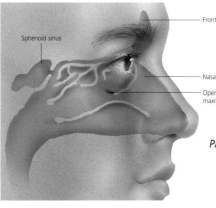

Sphenoid sinus
Frontal sinus
Nasal cavity
Opening of right maxillary sinus

Paranasal sinuses

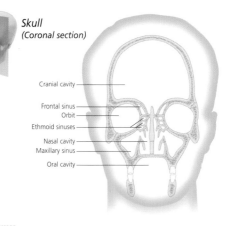

Skull (Sagittal section)

Frontal sinus
Ethmoid sinuses
Sphenoid sinus

Skull (Coronal section)

Cranial cavity
Frontal sinus
Orbit
Ethmoid sinuses
Nasal cavity
Maxillary sinus
Oral cavity

Normal   *Sinusitis*

Frontal sinus
Collected fluid in sinus
Maxillary sinus
Nasal septum
Nasal cavity
Narrowing of passage
Collected fluid in sinus

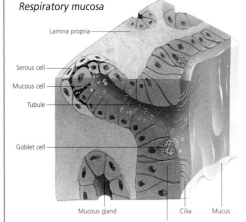

Respiratory mucosa

Lamina propria
Serous cell
Mucous cell
Tubule
Goblet cell
Mucous gland
Cilia
Mucus
Pseudostratified columnar epithelium

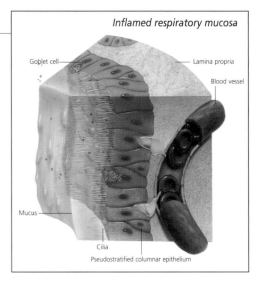

Inflamed respiratory mucosa

Goblet cell
Lamina propria
Blood vessel
Mucus
Cilia
Pseudostratified columnar epithelium

Symptoms of sinusitis

Sinusitis is usually indicated by the presence of thick, yellow- or green-colored nasal drainage, postnasal drip, cough, head congestion and headache. More specific symptoms of sinusitis vary depending on the type of sinusitis, the severity of the inflammation and the sinus cavities involved. If inadequately treated, sinusitis may last for months or years and involve the nose, eyes and middle ear. It is best to consult a physician promptly when any sinusitis symptoms appear.

Acute sinusitis – in addition to the presence of yellow or green pus, the most common symptoms of acute sinusitis are pain, tenderness and swelling around the affected sinus. Fever and chills may also be present.

    Maxillary sinusitis – pain in the cheekbone area under the eye; toothache; headache.

    Frontal sinusitis – headaches over the eyes or across the forehead.

    Ethmoid sinusitis – sharp pain between and behind the eyes; headache.

    Sphenoid sinusitis – typically more generalized, with pain in the front or back of the head.

Chronic sinusitis – symptoms of chronic sinusitis are usually less severe and painful than acute sinusitis. A feeling of nasal stuffiness, postnasal drip and decreased sense of smell are common. In addition, patients often feel generally unwell and/or fatigued.

Classification of sinusitis

Acute
Most often caused by a bacterial infection that develops after a viral respiratory illness (such as the common cold) and resulting sinus inflammation and blockage. May also result from a fungal infection, chronic nasal inflammation due to allergies, or underlying medical condition that has compromised the immune system. Symptoms last less than 4 weeks.

Subacute
A continuation of acute sinusitis symptoms that may be less severe (i.e., limited to congestion, headache or postnasal drip). Duration is usually 4 to 8 weeks.

Chronic
Sinusitis that lasts 8 to 12 consecutive weeks with varying degrees of severity. Can begin with an acute infection of the upper respiratory tract or be triggered by environmental causes (i.e., allergens or air pollution) or anatomical disorders, such as a deviated septum.

Recurrent
Three or more cases of acute sinusitis occurring within a 12-month period. May result from different infectious organisms at different times.

Inflammation and sinusitis

When the body is attacked by foreign microorganisms such as bacteria or viruses, a complex process called inflammation begins. Blood supply to the infected area is increased, and changes in blood vessel walls increase the amount of fluid and white blood cells delivered to the affected tissue. The heat, swelling, pain and fever commonly associated with infection are the result of the **immune response**, which targets the microorganisms with specialized cells and substances to limit the spread of infection and toxins. The immune system also produces pathogen-specific antibodies that immobilize and destroy the invading organisms. In sinusitis, inflammation in the nasal passages triggered by a cold or virus can block normal drainage of the sinuses. This allows the bacteria that normally live in the upper respiratory tract to multiply and cause infection.

Related sinus disease

Sinusitis may be caused or exacerbated by physical problems such as a deviated septum or nasal polyps, which interfere with normal sinus drainage. It may also be triggered by a fungal infection.

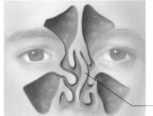

Deviated septum

What is a deviated septum?

The **nasal septum** is a thin layer of cartilage and bone that separates the nasal cavity into two passages (nostrils). If the septum is bent or deviated as a result of injury or birth defect, one nostril is often smaller and tighter than the other. A minor deviation in the septum usually goes unnoticed and does not produce any symptoms. More severe deviations can lead to breathing problems, nosebleeds or frequent inflammation of the sinuses, especially if drainage into the nasal cavity is blocked. A deviated septum can be corrected by surgery.

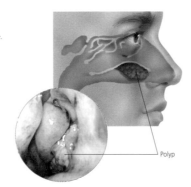

Polyp

What are nasal polyps?

Nasal polyps are small, fleshy, noncancerous growths that form on the mucous membranes of the nose, near the openings of the sinus cavities. They often do not produce specific symptoms, but patients with nasal polyps may be more prone to congestion, drainage problems and chronic sinus infections. Nasal polyps may be treated with medications or surgery.

What is allergic fungal sinusitis?

In patients with chronic sinus and rhinitis conditions or underlying immune problems, environmental fungi can trigger an allergic reaction involving significant nasal congestion and subsequent formation of nasal and sinus polyps. The inflammation and polyp growth are often limited to one side, and typically require surgery to remove debris and restore sinus drainage. Long-term medication therapy may be needed to eliminate the fungus and reduce inflammation.

Diagnosing and treating sinusitis

Diagnosis

Both chronic and acute sinusitis may have similar symptoms, including congestion and blocked sinus passages, facial pressure and pain, swelling, and tenderness. Infection in different sinus regions will produce specific symptoms, such as pain between the eyes in ethmoid sinusitis. Other general sinusitis symptoms (see above) used in diagnosis include yellow or green mucus, watery pus, red and swollen membranes, cough, loss of sense of smell, and bad breath.

Clinical diagnosis is often required to confirm the severity and exact location of a sinus infection. Your doctor may use a procedure called transillumination, in which a light source is held against the cheek to detect the presence of sinus fluid. Special 4-view x-rays and CT scans can also help pinpoint areas of swelling. In severe and chronic cases of sinusitis, other diagnostic procedures such as culture and sensitivity tests may also be necessary.

Treatment

A variety of treatment approaches are used to help relieve sinusitis pain and pressure as well as to improve drainage, reduce inflammation and clear infection. Common medication therapies include decongestants, antibiotics and corticosteroid nasal sprays. Length of antibiotic treatment can vary according to the severity of infection. For chronic or recurrent sinusitis, multiple courses of antibiotics may be required to completely clear the infection.

Other treatment approaches such as warm, moist heat applied to the face can also help to relieve sinus discomfort. Saline-based nasal washes are recommended by some practitioners to wash mucus and bacteria from the sinuses and maintain open nasal passages.

Long-term sinusitis that does not respond to antibiotic therapy may require surgery to clear drainage problems and improve breathing by removing excess and thickened mucous material and other debris in the sinus membranes.

PLATE 15

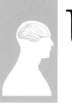

Understanding Depression

What is depression?

Depression is a significant change in mood that often involves feelings of intense sadness, hopelessness or disinterest in normal daily activities. After anxiety, depression is one of the most common mental health disorders in the United States and can interfere with the ability to work, sleep and eat. Depression may be triggered by traumatic life events or physical health problems and be prolonged or influenced by hereditary and other factors.

Types of depression

There are several types of depression. Depression that persists for more than two weeks is considered **major depression** and includes chronic symptoms such as depressed mood on most days, noticeable loss of pleasure in normal activities, loss of energy, sleeplessness and thoughts of suicide. In **chronic depression** (dysthymia), similar symptoms occur with less intensity but may last for a longer period of time. **Atypical depression** is characterized by excessive eating and sleeping behaviors and may occur simultaneously with other emotional disorders. **Seasonal affective disorder** (SAD) usually occurs during the winter months and is marked by fatigue, overeating and excess sleep patterns.

What causes depression?

There are multiple factors that can influence the onset, type and duration of depression, including environment, genetics, gender and biological factors such as physical illness.

Genetics
Research has shown that tendencies towards depression run in families, and genetics may be a factor in how likely patients are to develop the disorder.

Biological factors
Levels of brain chemicals such as serotonin play critical roles in feelings of well-being and have been strongly linked to depression. Other neurotransmitters such as dopamine and epinephrine may play an equally significant role in depression and anxiety.

Gender
Shifts in the female hormones estrogen and progesterone may strongly influence depressive episodes at various times through a woman's life.

Insomnia and sleep disorders
Insomnia may result from depression but can also be the cause of major changes in hormone activity leading to emotional problems. Changes in sleep patterns are known to exacerbate depression.

Depression risk factors

- Genetics/family history
- Medical conditions
- Drugs/toxins
- Loss and trauma

Depression symptoms

Depression is typically diagnosed when patients exhibit at least five of the following major depression symptoms (unrelated to acute episodes of grief or loss, alcohol or drug abuse, and cycles of manic behavior) for more than two weeks.

- Depressed mood
- Significant changes in appetite
- Insomnia
- Agitation
- Fatigue and loss of energy
- Frequent difficulty in concentrating
- Loss of pleasure in normal activities
- Significant weight gain
- Excessive sleeping
- Feeling of slowness
- Recurring sense of guilt/worthlessness
- Recurring thoughts of death or suicide

Depression is best diagnosed by a mental health specialist, such as a psychologist. There are several well-established screening tests that can help determine whether or not depression exists, as well as rule out other conditions and factors.

Synaptic cleft

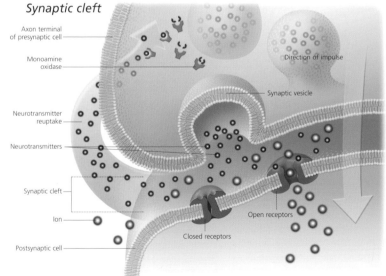

Axon terminal of presynaptic cell
Monoamine oxidase
Neurotransmitter reuptake
Neurotransmitters
Synaptic cleft
Ion
Closed receptors
Postsynaptic cell
Direction of impulse
Synaptic vesicle
Open receptors

Structure of the motor neuron

Direction of conduction
Dendrites
Myelin sheath (formed by Schwann cells)
Node of Ranvier
Axon
Nucleus
Nissl bodies (produce neurotransmitters)
Cell body
Direction of conduction
Telodendron
Synaptic knobs (or axon terminals of presynaptic neuron)
Direction of conduction

The cerebrum controls higher brain functions such as memory, speech and vision, while the cerebellum controls balance and coordination.

Frontal cortex
Corpus callosum
Thalamus
Hypothalamus
Ventral tegmental area
Optic chiasm
Pituitary gland
Mamillary body
Substantia nigra
Pons
Medulla oblongata
Cerebrum
Pineal gland
Cerebellum

What are synaptic connections?

The central nervous system (CNS) contains thousands of input and output connections between neurons that form dense networks within the brain. Synaptic connections are the tiny spaces between individual neurons where messenger chemicals called **neurotransmitters** bind to postsynaptic cell receptors which inhibit or excite electrical impulses within target cells. However, not all neurotransmitters bind to receptors. Neurotransmitters in the synaptic cleft may be degraded by enzymes or reabsorbed back into the axon terminal in a process called **reuptake**.

Norepinephrine pathways

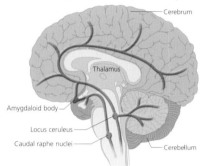

Cerebrum
Thalamus
Amygdaloid body
Locus ceruleus
Caudal raphe nuclei
Cerebellum

Serotonin pathways

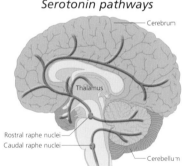

Cerebrum
Thalamus
Rostral raphe nuclei
Caudal raphe nuclei
Cerebellum

Neurotransmitter pathways

Neurotransmitters are highly specialized chemical messengers that carry impulses across tiny spaces between neurons (**nerve cells**) in the body. The impulses are sent by the axon of one presynaptic nerve cell and received by the dendrite of the postsynaptic cell. Neurotransmitters are secreted at the contact points between these cells (**synapses**) and trigger receptors on the dendrite to inhibit or excite neural impulses in the target cell. Each type of neurotransmitter (such as **dopamine** and **serotonin**) has unique characteristics that allow it to bind to specific receptor sites on target cells.

Taking control of your depression

Depression can be effectively managed and treated with a number of medications, as well as with cognitive behavioral therapy and other forms of psychotherapy. Lifestyle changes, dietary management (including vitamin supplementation) and exercise may also be very effective in improving mild to moderate depression.

The first step in taking control of depression is diagnosis by a qualified healthcare professional such as a psychologist. Depending on the type of depression, a number of options are available to help reduce the severity of symptoms and improve outlook and quality of life.

What is bipolar disorder?

Bipolar disorder is a complex illness that includes periods of depression and alternating periods of exaggerated euphoria or irritability known as mania. In most cases, the depressive cycles are much more frequent and longer-lasting than manic episodes. In some patients, however, both depression and mania exist at the same time. In all forms of bipolar disorder, the manifestations of the disease generally become more frequent and intense over time.

Depressive symptoms include lack of interest in formerly enjoyable activities; feelings of sadness or numbness; frequent episodes of crying; restlessness and irritability; appetite and weight changes; and difficulty concentrating or making decisions.

Manic symptoms can include irritability and anger; rapid thoughts and speech; insomnia; exaggerated sense of importance or power; and reckless behavior.

What causes bipolar disorder?

As in depression, a combination of factors is believed to be responsible for the chemical imbalances in the brain associated with the disease. Biologic factors may include abnormal activity in the parts of the brain that control emotion, concentration, inhibition and judgment. Family history (genetics) is also closely linked to the development of bipolar illness. Other possible causes currently under study are the influence of viruses and the interrelation of bipolar disorder with other illnesses such as schizophrenia, panic disorder and epilepsy.

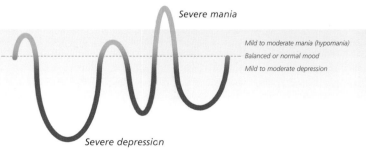

Severe mania
Mild to moderate mania (hypomania)
Balanced or normal mood
Mild to moderate depression
Severe depression

Bipolar disorder includes periods of depression and alternating periods of exaggerated euphoria or irritability known as mania.

PLATE 16

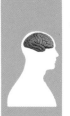

Understanding Migraines

What are migraines?

The term "migraine" is used to describe a recurring headache syndrome marked by acute sensitivity to environmental and sensory stimuli, such as light, sound, smells and movement. Physiological factors including hormonal fluctuations, excess stress or underlying conditions such as temporomandibular joint dysfunction can also trigger or exacerbate migraines. Considered a familial disease (tending to run in families), migraines typically affect three times as many women as men.

Migraine attacks are described as intense, throbbing pain on one or both sides of the head (pain can also begin on one side and switch to the other). The attacks can last anywhere from several hours to several days and recur as infrequently as once or twice a year or as often as several times weekly. Migraine attacks are often incapacitating and may be followed by a period of weakness and fatigue.

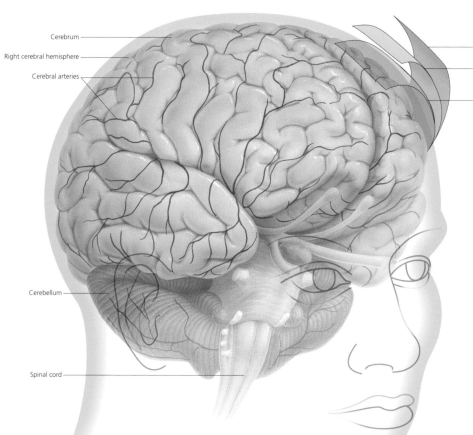

Cerebrum
Right cerebral hemisphere
Cerebral arteries
Cerebellum
Spinal cord

Meninges of the brain:
Dura mater
Arachnoid
Pia mater

Meninges of the brain

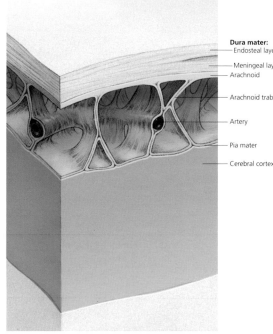

Dura mater:
Endosteal layer
Meningeal layer
Arachnoid
Arachnoid trabecula
Artery
Pia mater
Cerebral cortex

Arteriole

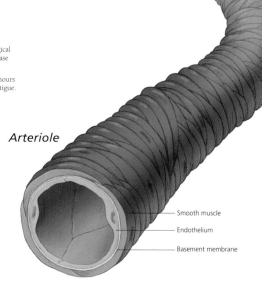

Smooth muscle
Endothelium
Basement membrane

Vasoconstriction

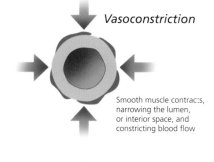

Smooth muscle contracts, narrowing the lumen, or interior space, and constricting blood flow

Vasodilation

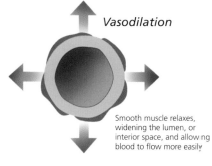

Smooth muscle relaxes, widening the lumen, or interior space, and allowing blood to flow more easily

Types of migraine headaches

There are two basic types of migraine headaches. **Migraine headache with aura** is preceded by a transient neurologic episode (aura), typically 20 minutes to an hour before the migraine begins. Auras can cause temporary visual disturbances such as tunnel vision, blind spots, flashing lights or shimmering zigzag lines. Auras may also temporarily affect balance, movement and speech. **Migraines without aura** (common migraine) develop gradually with no visual or sensory warning. They can also be present upon awakening. Migraines without aura are sometimes associated with prodromes, prolonged period of mood changes, food cravings, fluid retention and other symptoms that begin hours before onset of pain.

Migraine symptoms

Migraines can be distinguished from other types of headaches or head pain by the following clinical symptoms:

- Primarily unilateral pain (one side)
- Throbbing pain
- Acute sensitivity to light and sound
- Fluid retention
- Presence of an aura preceding the attack
- Moderate to severe pain
- Pain that worsens with movement
- Nausea and vomiting
- Mood changes

Depiction of a migraine aura

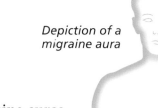

Serotonin pathways

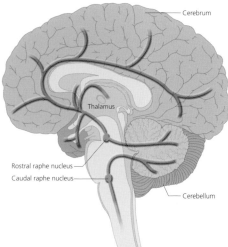

Cerebrum
Thalamus
Rostral raphe nucleus
Caudal raphe nucleus
Cerebellum

What causes migraine headaches?

While the exact cause of migraine headaches is not known, recent evidence suggests that a migraine attack originates as an electrical disturbance in the brain triggered by an outside source, such as food. These changes are believed to affect the release of **serotonin**, an important neurotransmitter that influences many functions in the brain, including pain thresholds and the constriction and dilation of blood vessels. As enlarged blood vessels trigger irritation in surrounding nerve endings, inflammation develops in the protective covering around the brain and spinal cord. The pain of migraine attacks is thought to result from a combination of increased pain sensitivity, vasodilation and inflammation.

Migraine auras

Migraine auras are temporary neurological events that affect one out of five migraine sufferers. They begin up to an hour before the onset of pain, and can include a variety of symptoms, including **visual disturbances** such as flashing lights, zigzag lines and luminous blind spots. **Non-visual aura symptoms**, including tingling, numbness and speech disturbances, may also occur, but are less common than visual auras.

Other events that can occur before and after a migraine are classified as **prodromes** and **postdromes**. Prodromes develop in approximately 50 percent of migraine patients, beginning up to 24 hours in advance of migraine pain. They are characterized by symptoms such as increased or diminished awareness, mood swings including irritability or depression, and food cravings. Postdromes last for 24 hours after migraine pain subsides, and most often include aching muscles and fatigue.

Migraine triggers

Identifying and avoiding individual triggers is a critical part of migraine management. Because triggers can include many different kinds of diet, medication, environmental and physiological stresses, it is important to keep a written diary listing potential triggers for each migraine attack, as well as the number and frequency of the attacks, responses to different treatments, and other details relevant to each attack.

Common dietary triggers
- Dairy products, particularly ripened cheese
- Fermented and pickled foods
- Alcohol and caffeine
- Processed meats
- Nuts and chocolate

Common environmental triggers
- Odors, including smoke and perfume
- Stress and time pressures
- Bright glare and flashing lights

Common physiological triggers
- Hormonal changes (menstrual periods and menopause)
- Excessive physical exertion
- Sleeping too much or too little
- Hunger or fasting

Synaptic cleft

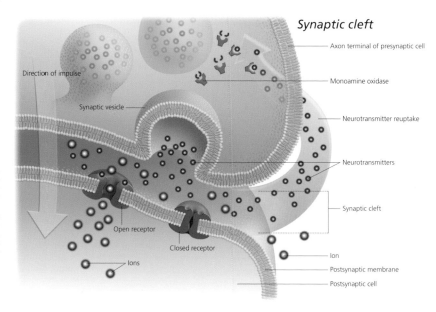

Direction of impulse
Synaptic vesicle
Open receptor
Closed receptor
Ions
Axon terminal of presynaptic cell
Monoamine oxidase
Neurotransmitter reuptake
Neurotransmitters
Synaptic cleft
Ion
Postsynaptic membrane
Postsynaptic cell

What are neurotransmitters?

Within the central nervous system (CNS) are dense networks of **neurons** (nerve cells) that send and receive signals via special "messenger" molecules called **neurotransmitters**. These highly specialized chemicals carry nerve impulses across the **synaptic gap**, a tiny space between the axon of a nerve cell and special receptor structures on the adjacent neurons.

Each neurotransmitter (for example, serotonin) has unique characteristics that allow it to bind to receptor sites on target cells and activate specific neural impulses. However, not all neurotransmitters are absorbed or used by target cells. Neurotransmitter molecules in the synaptic gap may be neutralized by enzyme degradation or reabsorbed back into the axon in a process called reuptake, which blocks the neurotransmitter's potential action.

Treatment options for migraines

Following a detailed physical exam and discussion of symptoms, migraine treatment frequently begins with the Migraine Disability Assessment Score (MIDAS) questionnaire, a clinical tool used to assess the degree of disability caused by migraine attacks and to help design an individualized migraine treatment approach. Because the effectiveness of different medications varies widely from one patient to another, a variety of over-the-counter and prescription drugs are often tried to identify those that combine the most effective and consistent relief with the fewest side effects. Nonmedicinal measures such as strict dietary guidelines to eliminate or reduce known triggers, lifestyle changes, stress reduction techniques and other approaches are also important components of successful treatment.

PLATE 17

Middle Ear Infections

Otitis media

Otitis media, commonly called a middle ear infection, is an inflammation of the **middle ear**. Otitis media is a common childhood illness with about 80% of children experiencing at least one episode by the age of four. Children and infants are prone to otitis media mainly because of immature **eustachian tubes** and immune systems.

There are different forms of otitis media with variations in symptoms, duration and treatments. The two most common categories are **acute otitis media** and **otitis media with effusion**. In both conditions, fluid, called effusion, usually collects in the middle ear space. This reduces the mobility of the tympanic membrane, often impairing hearing.

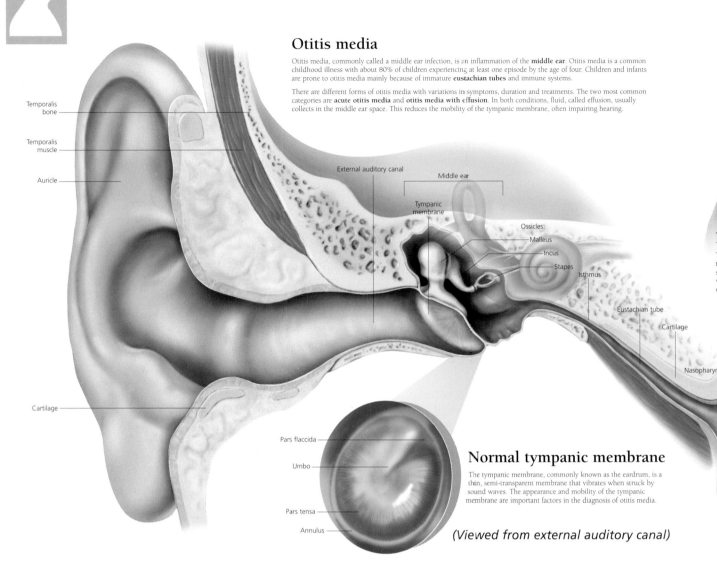

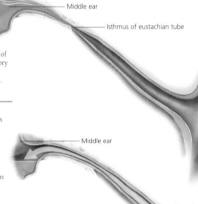

Middle ear

The middle ear is a small, air-filled cavity located behind the tympanic membrane that contains tiny bones called ossicles. The middle ear is connected to the respiratory system by the eustachian tube. The mucosal lining of the respiratory system is continuous with the lining of the eustachian tube and middle ear. This connection makes the middle ear susceptible to respiratory system inflammation and infection.

Eustachian tube in cross-section

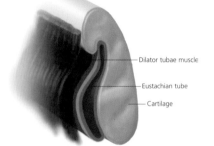

Normal tympanic membrane

The tympanic membrane, commonly known as the eardrum, is a thin, semi-transparent membrane that vibrates when struck by sound waves. The appearance and mobility of the tympanic membrane are important factors in the diagnosis of otitis media.

(Viewed from external auditory canal)

Eustachian tube

The eustachian tube normally lies flat but is opened by the dilator tubae muscle during yawning, sneezing and swallowing. When functioning properly, the eustachian tube performs three main functions:

- Ventilation of the middle ear by intermittent opening. This keeps middle-ear air pressure equal to outside air pressure.
- Drainage of middle ear secretions into the nasopharynx.
- Protection of the middle ear from nasopharyngeal secretions and sounds.

Acute otitis media

Acute otitis media is a painful middle ear inflammation in which effusion collects in the middle ear. It is characterized by a rapid onset of the symptoms of acute infection. The infection is usually caused by bacteria, although it can be viral.

Acute otitis media often follows an upper respiratory tract infection. Bacteria in the middle ear can proliferate in the effusion or can be aspirated into the middle ear from the nasopharynx.

If middle ear effusion persists for more than three months after an episode of acute otitis media, the condition becomes **chronic otitis media with effusion**.

Symptoms

Earache	Nausea and vomiting
Fever	Diarrhea
Hearing loss	Loss of appetite
Discharge from ear	Irritability

Bacteria

Streptococcus pneumoniae is the most common bacteria associated with acute otitis media.

Tympanic membrane
- Thickens and becomes opaque
- Appears full or bulging
- Lacks mobility

Eustachian tube dysfunction

Improper eustachian tube functioning is a common factor causing otitis media. Because children's eustachian tubes are not structurally or functionally mature, they are especially prone to these problems. Children's eustachian tubes are shorter and more horizontal than adults', allowing secretions from the nasopharynx to pass more easily into the middle ear. Due in part to having more flexible cartilage, the opening and closing mechanism of a child's eustachian tube often does not function properly.

Obstruction

Obstruction of the eustachian tube prevents middle ear secretions from draining into the nasopharynx, causing fluid to accumulate in the middle ear. The tube can become blocked because of allergies or enlarged tonsils, but often the culprit is an upper respiratory tract infection. The respiratory mucosa becomes congested, and the narrowest part of the eustachian tube, the **isthmus**, becomes blocked.

Aspiration

Secretions in the nasopharynx, often containing bacteria, can be aspirated up the eustachian tube and into the middle ear. Two reasons that aspiration of fluid can occur:

- The eustachian tube stays open, allowing secretions to flow into the middle ear. Lying horizontally makes it easier for the fluid to reach the middle ear.
- The eustachian tube does not open properly, so air pressure in the middle ear cannot be regulated. A negative pressure is created within the middle ear, which pulls the fluid from the nasopharynx up the eustachian tube.

Treatments

The treatment of otitis media varies according to the type, severity and duration of the condition. Sometimes active treatments are not necessary, and watchful waiting is the most appropriate course of action.

Antibiotics

Your doctor will often prescribe a course of antibiotics to eliminate any bacterial infection in the middle ear or respiratory system. There is currently a new series of vaccines for preventing the most common causes of middle ear infections.

Surgical management

Myringotomy and tympanostomy tube insertion can be used to ventilate and drain an effusion in the middle ear. The myringotomy can be performed as a separate procedure or in conjunction with the insertion of a tympanostomy tube.

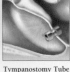

Myringotomy
An incision is made in the tympanic membrane.

Tympanostomy Tube
A tympanostomy tube is inserted into the incision.

Otitis media with effusion

Otitis media with effusion is an inflammatory condition in which fluid collects in the middle ear, but there are no symptoms of acute infection. Otitis media can occur in conjunction with an upper respiratory tract infection, after an episode of acute otitis media, or independent of other illnesses. Bacteria may or may not be present in the effusion.

Otitis media with effusion differs from acute otitis media in that it is generally a painless condition. For this reason, otitis media with effusion may be present for a long time before being diagnosed.

Otitis media with effusion often resolves spontaneously without treatment. If the effusion fails to resolve after a reasonable amount of time, surgical management may be indicated.

Symptoms

Otitis media with effusion can be asymptomatic, but if symptoms are present, they are often vague. Mild to moderate hearing loss and a feeling of fullness or ringing in the ear are most common.

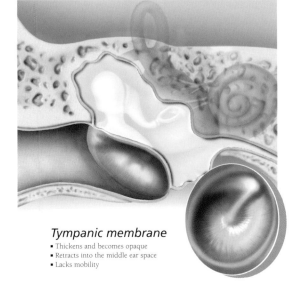

Tympanic membrane
- Thickens and becomes opaque
- Retracts into the middle ear space
- Lacks mobility

Ruptured tympanic membrane

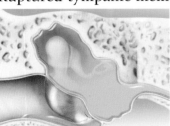

As a result of pressure effusion from acute otitis media in the middle ear, the tympanic membrane can spontaneously rupture. This opening allows drainage of fluid or pus from the middle ear into the external auditory canal and eustachian tube. The perforation generally closes within 3 weeks.

PLATE 18

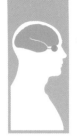

Understanding Glaucoma

What is glaucoma?

Glaucoma is a group of diseases in which the normal pressure of the fluid inside the eyes (intraocular pressure) is increased. This can lead to loss of vision and, possibly, to blindness if the condition is left untreated. Glaucoma affects about 1 in 20 people at the age of 70 years. It is more common and may be more severe in black people and in people with a family history of the disease. The most common form of the disease is open angle glaucoma, which affects about two-thirds of glaucoma sufferers.

There is a small space at the front of the eye called the **anterior chamber**. The **ciliary body** supports the lens and produces a watery fluid, the **aqueous humor**, which bathes and nourishes the neighboring tissues. The aqueous humor is drained constantly through a spongy mesh that lies in the angle between the **iris** and the inner surface of the **cornea**. The fluid drains too slowly in people with open angle glaucoma. This causes the intraocular pressure to increase and the cornea to swell. These changes can result in damage to the **optic nerve**. The optic nerve connects the light-sensitive **retina** to the brain and any damage to it can result in defects in vision.

At first, people with glaucoma are free of symptoms. Vision is normal, and there is no pain associated with the condition. As the disease progresses, people may have difficulty moving from a bright room into a darker one and in judging steps and curbs. A person with glaucoma may continue to see objects directly in front of him clearly. However, objects to the side (periphery) may be missed. Blindness can result from a progressive loss of visual field if the disease remains untreated.

The cause of glaucoma

Fluid normally passes through a narrow space between the iris and lens, then drains out of the eye through the **scleral venous sinus**. If this outward flow is blocked, pressure can damage the optic nerve and reduce vision.

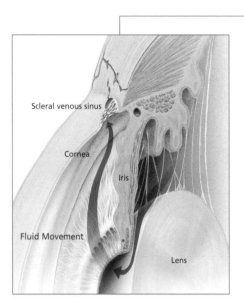

Scleral venous sinus
Cornea
Iris
Fluid Movement
Lens

The structure of the eye

The wall of the eyeball is made up of three layers. The outermost layer, the **fibrous tunic**, contains both the **sclera** (gives shape to the eyeball) and the **cornea** (transmits and refracts light). The middle layer, the **vascular tunic**, is made up of the **choroid** (supplies blood to the eye), the **ciliary body** (supports the **lens** and produces a fluid called the **aqueous humor**) and the **iris** (regulates the amount of light by controlling **pupil** size). The innermost layer, the **internal tunic**, contains the **retina** (provides photoreception and transmits impulses). Within the eyeball and suspended from the ciliary body by the **suspensory ligament** is the lens, which refracts and focuses the light onto the retina.

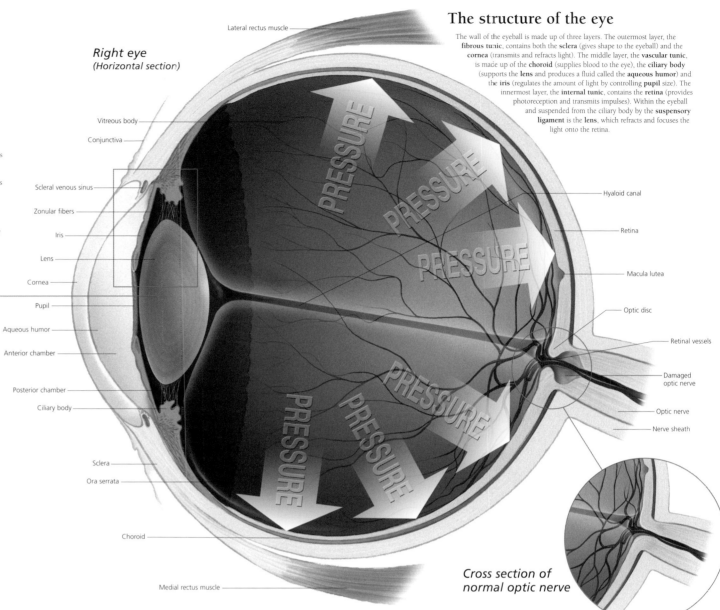

Right eye
(Horizontal section)

Lateral rectus muscle
Vitreous body
Conjunctiva
Scleral venous sinus
Zonular fibers
Iris
Lens
Cornea
Pupil
Aqueous humor
Anterior chamber
Posterior chamber
Ciliary body
Sclera
Ora serrata
Choroid
Medial rectus muscle

Hyaloid canal
Retina
Macula lutea
Optic disc
Retinal vessels
Damaged optic nerve
Optic nerve
Nerve sheath

PRESSURE

Cross section of normal optic nerve

How is glaucoma diagnosed?

Glaucoma is a chronic disease that develops slowly. Damage to the optic nerve and visual loss have developed in many patients before the condition has been diagnosed. Regular eye examinations are essential in people who are at risk of developing glaucoma and in those who have been diagnosed with the disease.

A range of tests are used to diagnose and monitor glaucoma:

Visual acuity
The ability of the person to see at various distances is measured using eye charts. These usually consist of letters of different sizes against a plain background.

Tonometry
It has been known for over 100 years that the assessment of intraocular pressure is important in the diagnosis and monitoring of glaucoma. However, it has been recognized more recently that there is no cutoff point between normal and raised intraocular pressure. High intraocular pressure increases a person's risk of developing glaucoma but it does not mean that the person has the disease. The development of glaucoma in an individual depends upon the level of intraocular pressure that the optic nerve will tolerate.

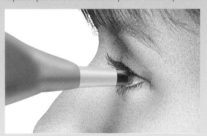

Applanation tonometer

Tonometry is a term used to describe the methods of measuring intraocular pressure. There are many different types of tonometry. The Goldmann applanation tonometer subjects the eye to sufficient force to flatten the cornea. The force applied is measured using a cobalt blue light source and is related to the intraocular pressure by a mathematical equation.

Another type of tonometry relates the time required to flatten the cornea using a puff of air to the intraocular pressure. This method is useful in screening people for glaucoma.

Pupil dilation
Drops are put into the eye to widen the pupil. This allows signs of damage to the optic nerve to be observed more easily.

Visual field
Peripheral vision is measured using the technique of perimetry. The test involves illuminated targets being projected onto an illuminated background. The brightness of the targets is varied so that the average luminescence of the dimmest target can be calculated. The test is repeated several times within the visual field, and any abnormalities are detected using a computer printout.

Perimetry is used to show the extent of any damage due to glaucoma and also to check on any progression of the disease.

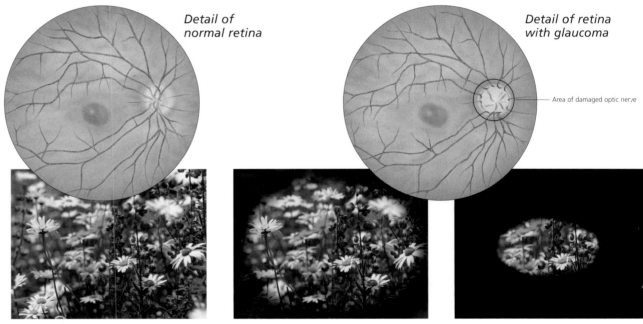

Detail of normal retina

Detail of retina with glaucoma

Area of damaged optic nerve

Field of vision loss
The sequence of photographs suggests the progressive narrowing of the field of vision characteristic of glaucoma.

How is glaucoma treated?

The best way to control glaucoma is to ensure that it is detected and treated as early as possible. People who fall into high-risk groups should have their eyes examined regularly. It is essential that people with glaucoma have their condition monitored at regular intervals.

Glaucoma cannot be cured, but it can be corrected in most people. A variety of treatments can be used, depending on the severity of the condition.

Most people with open angle glaucoma are treated with medications. The most common initial treatment is eye drops containing a beta-blocker, such as timolol. These lower the intraocular pressure by reducing the production of aqueous humor and delay the progress of glaucoma. Some people are unable to tolerate beta-blockers or have other medical conditions that prevent their use. Dorzolamide or brinzolamide also reduce the production of aqueous humor and may be suitable for these people. They can also be used in combination with beta-blockers. Other eye drops, such as adrenaline or pilocarpine, can be added as necessary to control intraocular pressure. Apraclonidine is a drug that lowers the intraocular pressure by reducing the rate of production of aqueous humor. Latanoprost lowers the intraocular pressure by increasing the drainage of the aqueous humor from the anterior chamber.

Medication will control intraocular pressure in most people with glaucoma. However, it is essential that medication is used regularly and that glaucoma is monitored to ensure that the combination of drugs selected remains effective.

In some people, medication may not be effective in controlling glaucoma, and surgical treatments have to be considered. In laser surgery, a strong beam of light is focused on the part of the anterior chamber where the aqueous humor is drained from the eye. Changes in the tissue following exposure to the laser result in improved drainage of the aqueous fluid from the eye. The effects of laser surgery may wear off with time. Medication is continued in many patients to maintain long-term benefits.

Surgery is usually reserved for people whose intraocular pressure cannot be controlled by medication or laser surgery. A channel is created in the eye so that the aqueous humor can leave the eye more easily, and intraocular pressure is reduced. Medication is usually required following surgery.

PLATE 19

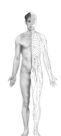

Understanding Parkinson's Disease

What is Parkinson's disease?

Parkinson's disease is a slow, degenerative disorder of the nervous system that is characterized by tremors, slow movement and rigid muscle tone. It results from the development of lesions in the basal nuclei (or extrapyramidal circuit), an area of the brain that works in harmony with the motor cortex (pyramidal system) and is responsible for initiating and coordinating voluntary movement. These lesions interfere with the synthesis and release of dopamine, a neurotransmitter that allows signals for movement to be relayed from the brain to the muscles.

Parkinson's disease typically begins between the ages of 40 and 70 and is one of the most common causes of disability among older people. Onset is usually very gradual. It may be difficult to pinpoint the appearance of initial symptoms, which may be mild or appear only during a period of stress, followed by months or years of remission.

Risk factors for Parkinson's disease

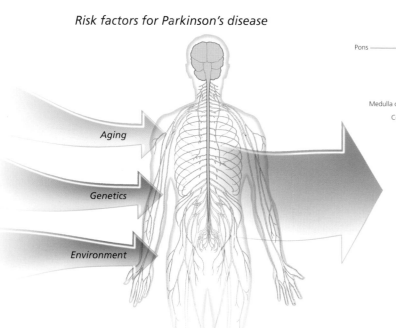

Aging

Genetics

Environment

What causes Parkinson's disease?

While the exact cause of Parkinson's disease has not been clearly established, a combination of genetic and environmental risk factors has been associated with development of the disease.

- **AGING** Risks of developing Parkinson's disease appear to increase with each decade, and aging itself may contribute to a decrease in dopamine-producing neurons. However, there is no clear evidence that links age as a cause of the disease.
- **GENETICS** Six genes have been identified that may play a key role in development of Parkinson's disease, including the Parkin gene. Ongoing research on genetic risk factors will hopefully lead to improved diagnosis and treatment.
- **ENVIRONMENT** There are multiple theories linking Parkinson's disease with exposure to environmental toxins, particularly pesticides. Welding has also been identified as a potential environmental risk factor.

Symptoms of Parkinson's disease

The four cardinal signs of Parkinson's disease are:

- **TREMOR** The first indication of disease in many patients, tremor may be present in one or more limbs, usually when the limb is at rest (but not during sleep). Tremors often involve a back-and-forth or shaking type of motion. A common type of tremor is a "pill rolling" movement of the fingers and thumb.
- **RIGIDITY** Muscle rigidity and stiffness result in a loss of mobility and make it difficult to carry out simple tasks involving fine motor skills, such as writing or tying shoes. Rigidity impairs walking, and can cause a shuffling gait or sudden immobility. Over time, rigidity may affect the facial muscles, creating a lack of expression, and undermine functions such as swallowing or speaking.
- **BRADYKINESIA/AKINESIA** Both terms refer to movement that is slow, limited in scope, or lacking in spontaneity. It becomes difficult to start or stop movement and reaction times are noticeably slow.
- **POSTURAL INSTABILITY** One of the later symptoms of Parkinson's disease, postural instability is caused by lack of balance combined with stooped posture, creating a tendency to fall forward.

Secondary symptoms that develop in some but not all patients include:

- Soft, monotonal speech
- Gastrointestinal problems; swallowing or constipation
- Abnormal sleepiness and other sleep problems
- Blurred vision and fixed gaze
- Loss of libido
- Depression, dementia and other cognitive disturbances
- Lightheadedness (orthostatic hypotension)
- Loss of smell and taste
- Increased sweating
- Urinary dysfunction

The brain
(Coronal section)

Motor cortex

Cerebrum

Corticospinal pathway (pyramidal system)

Basal nuclei (extrapyramidal system)
- Caudate nucleus
- Putamen
- Globus pallidus

Thalamus

Pons

Medulla oblongota

Cerebellum

From sensory cell in muscle

To lower motor neurons

How is normal movement produced?

The body's ability to produce and direct movement is controlled by a complex motor pathway involving two separate systems. The **pyramidal system** extends from the motor cortex in the brain to the spinal cord, which transmits signals to the muscles. The **extrapyramidal circuit** (also called the basal nuclei) modulates the activity of the pyramidal system. It encompasses 5 distinct areas in the brain and relies on the production of dopamine by neurons in the substantia nigra to initiate or inhibit movement appropriately.

Dopamine pathways

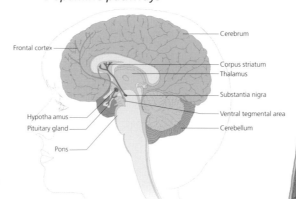

Frontal cortex

Cerebrum

Corpus striatum

Thalamus

Substantia nigra

Hypothalamus

Pituitary gland

Ventral tegmental area

Cerebellum

Pons

The role of dopamine

Dopamine is a neurotransmitter produced by specialized neurons of the **substantia nigra**, a portion of the brain located within the basal ganglia. Dopamine regulates fine motor coordination, thought, short-term memory and many other critical body functions. The symptoms of Parkinson's disease develop when a large percentage of dopamine-producing neurons degenerate, altering the normal processes that stimulate as well as inhibit motion.

Cerebrum

Pons

Medulla oblongota

Cerebellum

Spinal cord

Ganglion

Superficial branch of the radial nerve

Ulnar nerve

Median nerve

Digital nerve

Synaptic cleft

Monoamine oxidase

Axon terminal of presynaptic cell

Synaptic vesicle

Dopamine

Reuptake of dopamine

Synaptic cleft

Dopamine receptor site

Postsynaptic cell

Open

Closed

Receptors

Ion

What are synaptic connections?

The central nervous system (CNS) contains thousands of input and output connections between neurons that form dense networks within the brain. Synaptic connections are the tiny spaces between individual neurons where neurotransmitters are exchanged, initiating new electrical currents within target cells.

Neurotransmitters such as dopamine are highly specialized chemical messengers that carry impulses across tiny spaces between **neurons** (nerve cells) in the brain. The impulses are sent by the axon of one nerve cell and received by the dendrite of the next. Neurotransmitters are secreted at the contact points between these cells (**synapses**) and trigger receptors on the dendrite to activate or inhibit neural impulses. There are at least 6 different forms of dopamine receptors, each playing a slightly different role in stimulating and inhibiting movement.

Like other neurotransmitters, dopamine molecules that are not absorbed or used by target cells are neutralized through enzyme degradation or reabsorbed back into the axon terminal in a process called **reuptake**, where they may be stored again for later release.

Stages of Parkinson's disease

The Hoehn and Yahr scale uses 5 general stages to classify the severity of Parkinson's disease. Patients may not experience symptoms in this order.

Stage I: Symptoms affect one side of the body and typically include tremors and **bradykinesia** (slowness of movement) as well as visible changes in muscle tone, posture and balance.

Stage II: Symptoms are more advanced, affecting both sides of the body, and may include difficulty walking, speech abnormalities and problems completing everyday tasks.

Stage III: More severe symptoms affect the ability to walk or stand. Movement is noticeably slow, though patients still function independently.

Stage IV: Patients have severe difficulty performing normal activities and can no longer live independently.

Stage V: Patients are unable to walk or get out of bed and require a wheelchair.

Diagnosing and treating Parkinson's disease

Diagnosis

Early Parkinson's disease is often difficult to diagnose, especially in older patients with similar age-related symptoms, such as slow movement or muscle stiffness. In many cases, diagnosis is made after re-examination over several months. Once Parkinson's has been identified, further clinical diagnosis must be conducted to rule out other parkinsonian-type disorders. Combination of symptoms, speed of disease progression and response to medication therapy are key to clinical diagnosis. Neuroimaging (CT or MRI scans) may also be used.

Treatment

The two primary approaches to treatment are **physical activity** and **drug therapy**. Patients are encouraged to maintain an active daily routine as long as possible, including regular exercise and physical and occupational therapy focused on maintaining muscle tone, range of motion and independence.

The goal of drug therapy is to control symptoms and enhance movement for as long as possible while minimizing unwanted complications such as motor fluctuations ("on" and "off" cycles, characterized by alternating periods of "freezing" and mobility) and **dyskinesia** (sudden uncontrollable movement). Choices and doses of different drugs, such as dopamine precursors that stimulate the brain to produce additional dopamine, are individually tailored based on age, health, severity and progression of symptoms and response to therapy. Other drugs may be used to control non-motor symptoms of Parkinson's disease, such as gastrointestinal or cognitive/psychiatric disturbances.

PLATE 20

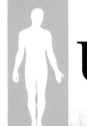

Understanding the Prostate

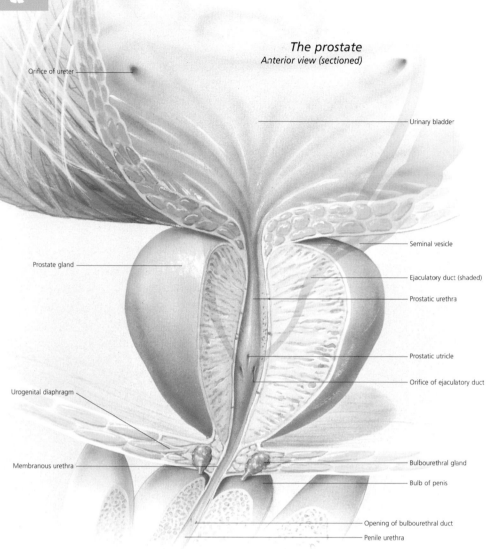

The prostate
Anterior view (sectioned)

Orifice of ureter

Prostate gland

Urogenital diaphragm

Membranous urethra

Urinary bladder

Seminal vesicle

Ejaculatory duct (shaded)

Prostatic urethra

Prostatic utricle

Orifice of ejaculatory duct

Bulbourethral gland

Bulb of penis

Opening of bulbourethral duct

Penile urethra

What is the prostate?

The prostate is a small gland located beneath the bladder and just in front of the rectum, behind the base of the penis. The prostate is similar to a walnut in both shape and size and surrounds the upper portion of the **urethra**, which passes through it. The primary purpose of the prostate is the production of fluid for semen. It also functions as a valve, preventing the leakage of urine from the bladder and the entry of sperm and seminal fluid into the bladder.

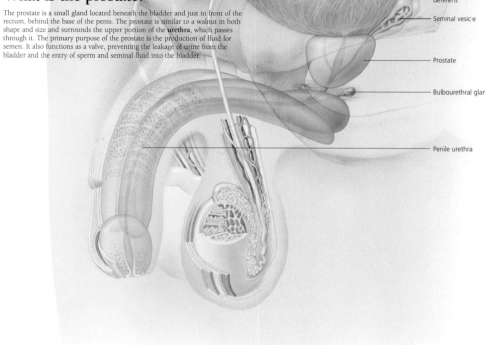

Ureter

Ductus deferens

Bladder

Ampulla of ductus deferens

Seminal vesicle

Prostate

Bulbourethral gland

Penile urethra

Prostate — zones
Sagittal section

Zones of the prostate

There are three primary zones within the prostate. The outermost section is called the **peripheral zone**. It makes up approximately 70% of the prostate gland's total volume and is the area where prostate cancer is most likely to develop. The innermost section of the prostate is the **transition zone**, a small area that surrounds the urethra. In **benign prostatic hyperplasia** or BPH (see below), noncancerous growth of tissue (hyperplasia) in the transition zone causes constriction of the urethra and restricts urinary flow. Between these two zones is the **central zone** of the prostate, through which the ejaculatory ducts pass.

Zone key:
- Central zone
- Peripheral zone
- Transition zone
- Anterior zone

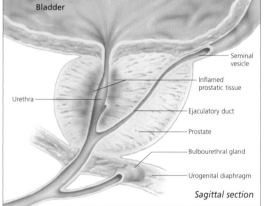

Bladder

Seminal vesicle

Inflamed prostatic tissue

Urethra

Ejaculatory duct

Prostate

Bulbourethral gland

Urogenital diaphragm

Sagittal section

What is prostatitis?

Prostatitis is a painful condition involving infection or inflammation of the prostate gland. The most common of all prostate diseases, its symptoms include pain between the rectum and testicles, in the groin and genital area, and in the lower back. There are several types of prostatitis, including **acute** and **chronic**, **bacterial** and **nonbacterial**. It is typically diagnosed by urinalysis and treated with antibiotics, anti-inflammatory drugs, and other medications. Unfortunately, the causes of chronic prostatitis, the most common form of the disease, are not yet understood. Research into improved treatments for prostatitis is ongoing.

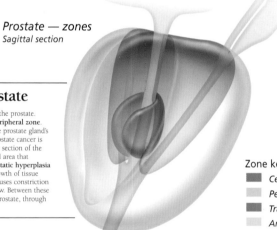

Bladder

Prostatic urethra

Prostate

Cancerous tumor

Sagittal section

Detection and treatment of prostate cancer

Recent improvements in detection methods are now allowing earlier diagnosis and treatment of prostate cancer. This has produced a significant decline in mortality rates in recent years.

Symptoms

Although early stages of prostate cancer often go unnoticed, a variety of symptoms may occur as the disease progresses. Many of these symptoms are also associated with benign prostatic hyperplasia (BPH), a noncancerous condition.
- Frequent urination, particularly at night
- Inability to urinate or difficulty starting urination
- Pain or burning during urination
- Presence of blood in urine or semen
- Difficulty achieving an erection
- Pain during ejaculation
- Chronic pain or stiffness in the lower back or legs

What is benign prostatic hyperplasia (BPH)?

BPH, also known as **enlarged prostate**, is a noncancerous growth of tissue within the transition zone that can restrict urination and cause other urinary problems. It is a common condition in men over 60 years of age. BPH is **not associated with prostate cancer** and can be effectively treated. About one third of all men with BPH will eventually require treatment for their symptoms.

BPH symptoms and treatment

BPH symptoms include a **weak urine stream**, a sensation of **incomplete emptying** of the bladder, **urinary frequency** and **urgency**, and the need to **urinate several times during the night**.

Diagnosis of BPH is based on factors including medical history, a physical exam, and a symptom score assessment. **Blood tests**, **urinalysis**, **X-rays**, **cystoscopy**, **ultrasound** and other tests may be used to confirm the diagnosis and guide treatment decisions.

Treatment options include:
- **Watchful waiting** — if symptoms are manageable
- **Medication therapy** — to relax the prostate muscles, shrink prostatic tissue, or both
- **Minimally invasive therapies** — such as microwave thermotherapy heat targeted areas of prostate tissue to relieve symptoms
- **TURP** — or transurethral resection of the prostate involves the surgical removal of the inner portion of the prostate
- **Phytotherapeutics** — saw palmetto and other plant-based therapies may be effective in treating BPH but are not FDA approved

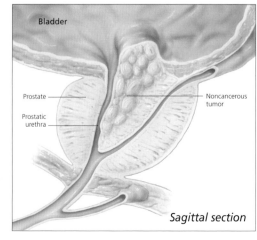

Bladder

Prostate

Prostatic urethra

Noncancerous tumor

Sagittal section

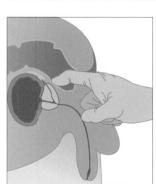

Digital rectal exam

Detection

The most reliable detection of early prostate cancer involves a combination of two tests:
- **Digital rectal exam** — a physical examination of the prostate via the rectum. It detects hardness, bumps, or swelling caused by cancer or other prostate problems. While this test is important, it often cannot detect prostate cancer until it is more advanced.
- **Prostate specific antigen (PSA)** — a blood test that measures an enzyme produced by the prostate. An elevated PSA is considered the best predictor of prostate cancer and can detect the presence of disease up to 6 years earlier than a digital rectal exam.

If either test indicates a possibility of cancer, additional tests may be performed to confirm the diagnosis:
- **Transrectal ultrasonography** — to measure prostate size and locate possible sites of cancer cells for needle biopsy.
- **Needle biopsy** — tissue samples are taken from several areas of the prostate for microscopic diagnosis.

Treatment

The type of treatment recommended varies from patient to patient. A classification method called the **Gleason score** is often used to rank malignancy and determine the most appropriate treatment.
- **Watchful waiting** — recommended for some men with early, slow-growing prostate cancer or other serious medical problems.
- **Surgery** — options for more advanced disease include radical prostatectomy (removal of the entire prostate gland) and nerve-sparing surgery, a newer surgical technique.
- **Radiation** — external beam radiation therapy offers a highly effective alternative to surgery in many prostate cancer patients.
- **Brachytherapy** — radioactive seeds are implanted in the prostate to eradicate cancer cells.
- **Hormone therapy** — generally recommended when prostate cancer has spread to other tissues. Hormones linked to the growth of cancer cells are inhibited through surgical or drug therapy.

PLATE 21

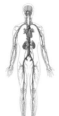

Understanding Metabolic Syndrome

What is metabolic syndrome?

Metabolic syndrome is a group of dangerous health disorders that work together to increase the risk of cardiovascular disease. Closely linked to a condition known as insulin resistance, metabolic syndrome is also known as **syndrome X, diabesity** and **dysmetabolic syndrome**.

Although the exact cause of metabolic syndrome is not known, it is believed to be a combination of lifestyle/activity, diet and genetic factors. The most important characteristics of metabolic syndrome include high triglyceride levels, high blood pressure, low HDL and high LDL cholesterol levels, abdominal obesity and high blood glucose.

The precursors of metabolic syndrome can begin in childhood, and the risks continue to increase with age. Many people are diagnosed with metabolic syndrome in their sixties and seventies. At present, nearly 50 million adults in the U.S. are estimated to have metabolic syndrome.

How is metabolic syndrome diagnosed?

Among the diagnostic measurements listed below, insulin resistance and the distribution of abdominal fat are considered key indicators for diagnosing metabolic syndrome. Additional criteria continue to be defined as more is learned about the condition.

- Waistline measurements exceeding 40 inches for men or 36 inches for women
- Blood pressure above 130/85 mm HG
- Triglyceride levels exceeding 150 mg/dL
- Fasting blood glucose levels higher than 100 mg/dL
- HDL (high density lipoprotein) levels below 40 mg/dL (men) or 50 mg/dL (women)

Beyond these considerations, three specific patient groups are often associated with metabolic syndrome:
- Diabetics who cannot maintain proper glucose levels
- Non-diabetics with high blood pressure and elevated blood glucose levels
- Patients with previous heart attacks who secrete high levels of insulin but are not glucose intolerant

Environmental factors — *Genetic factors*

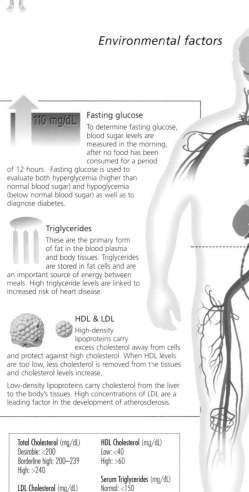

Fasting glucose
110 mg/dL
To determine fasting glucose, blood sugar levels are measured in the morning, after no food has been consumed for a period of 12 hours. Fasting glucose is used to evaluate both hyperglycemia (higher than normal blood sugar) and hypoglycemia (below normal blood sugar) as well as to diagnose diabetes.

Triglycerides
These are the primary form of fat in the blood plasma and body tissues. Triglycerides are stored in fat cells and are an important source of energy between meals. High triglyceride levels are linked to increased risk of heart disease.

HDL & LDL
High-density lipoproteins carry excess cholesterol away from cells and protect against high cholesterol. When HDL levels are too low, less cholesterol is removed from the tissues and cholesterol levels increase.

Low-density lipoproteins carry cholesterol from the liver to the body's tissues. High concentrations of LDL are a leading factor in the development of atherosclerosis.

Blood pressure
The force exerted by the blood against the walls of the blood vessels is known as blood pressure. It is directly affected by how hard the heart is beating, the amount of blood in the body and the diameter of the blood vessels. High blood pressure refers to abnormally high pressure in the arteries, which can damage the vessel walls if untreated.

Abdominal obesity
40
Excess fat (adipose) tissue accumulation in the abdomen is associated with significant risk of metabolic syndrome and related health problems, including abnormal lipid levels. Simple waist measurement used to assess abdominal fat content is considered a more sensitive indicator of risk than Body Mass Index (BMI), even in patients with overall obesity.

Total Cholesterol (mg/dL)	HDL Cholesterol (mg/dL)
Desirable: <200	Low: <40
Borderline high: 200–239	High: >60
High: >240	
LDL Cholesterol (mg/dL)	**Serum Triglycerides (mg/dL)**
Optimal: <100	Normal: <150
Near/above optimal: 100–129	Borderline high: 150–199
Borderline high: 130–159	High: 200–499
High: 160–189	Very High: >500
Very high: >190	

Stroke

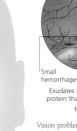

Hemorrhagic stroke
Area of burst arterioles

Ischemic stroke
Embolus or blockage of arteries

When an artery supplying the brain with oxygen becomes blocked by a blood clot or fat deposits, blood supply can be severely restricted, causing a stroke. Strokes can also occur as a result of the rupture of a bulging artery (aneurysm).

Arteries that have become narrowed as a result of atherosclerosis or other conditions limit blood flow to the brain, potentially leading to stroke. Smoking, diabetes and high blood pressure are all contributing factors to the development of atherosclerosis.

Retina — Healthy vessels

Small hemorrhages

Exudates (accumulations of protein that have leaked out)

Narrowing of arteries

Vision problems are a common side effect of diabetes, specifically a condition known as retinopathy. In this eye complication, the small blood vessels that supply the retina with blood weaken and leak, damaging the retina and hindering its ability to transmit images to the brain. Diabetics also have an increased risk for glaucoma and cataracts.

What is insulin resistance?

Insulin is an important hormone that helps to control the metabolism of the foods we eat and the levels of glucose in the blood. In metabolic syndrome, the body's cells become resistant to the normal effects of insulin and do not absorb glucose from the blood properly to use for energy. The pancreas compensates by secreting additional insulin. In some people, inability to process glucose efficiently allows glucose levels to build up in the bloodstream, raising cholesterol and triglyceride levels and causing coronary artery damage as well as leading to the onset of type 2 diabetes.

Action of Insulin

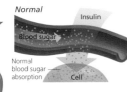

Normal
Insulin
Blood sugar
Normal blood sugar absorption
Cell

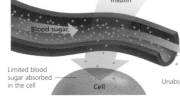

Insulin resistant
Insulin
Blood sugar
Limited blood sugar absorbed in the cell
Cell
Unabsorbed blood sugars

Insulin

Blood Glucose Level

Glucagon
Epinephrine Cortisol
Human Growth Hormone

Function of insulin
During digestion, sugar is absorbed into the bloodstream and stimulates the production of insulin in the pancreas. Insulin allows glucose to diffuse from the blood into essential body tissues, particularly the skeletal muscles. Insulin also controls blood sugar by promoting protein synthesis in the cells and regulating glucose and glycogen conversion in the liver.

Insulin resistance and type 2 diabetes
Type 2 diabetes is closely related to obesity and occurs when the body becomes resistant to the normal effects of insulin. The pancreas continues to produce insulin, but not in sufficient quantities to meet the body's needs. Type 2 diabetes can also occur as a result of a partial failure of the pancreas.

Effects of metabolic syndrome

Metabolic syndrome can result in a variety of serious health problems linked to the central disorder of insulin resistance. Over time, high levels of insulin and glucose in the blood can damage the blood vessel linings and increase the risks of blood clot formation, heart disease and stroke. Kidney function can be impaired, increasing blood pressure and increasing cardiovascular risks. Metabolic syndrome is closely associated with the onset of type 2 diabetes, which can damage the eyes, nerves and kidneys.

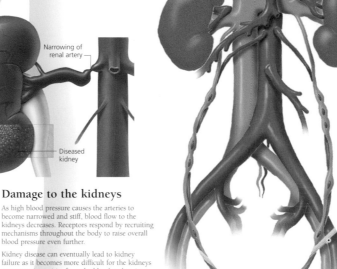

Normal artery

Artery with plaque

Ruptured plaque

Blocked artery

Damage to blood vessels

Artery walls become damaged as a result of untreated high blood pressure and accumulation of fats that cause the walls to thicken. As calcium is deposited in the fatty areas, "hardening" occurs and restricts the arteries from increasing in size. Damaged artery walls may also cause blood clots to form, blocking the artery itself or breaking away and blocking arteries in other organs.

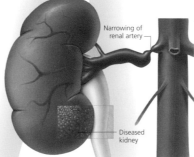

Narrowing of renal artery

Diseased kidney

Damage to the kidneys

As high blood pressure causes the arteries to become narrowed and stiff, blood flow to the kidneys decreases. Receptors respond by recruiting mechanisms throughout the body to raise overall blood pressure even further.

Kidney disease can eventually lead to kidney failure as it becomes more difficult for the kidneys to remove impurities from the blood and toxic materials accumulate.

Diet and lifestyle changes

The keys to managing metabolic syndrome are to address its underlying causes: physical inactivity and excess weight. Treatment focuses on losing weight to restore the body's ability to process insulin and on increasing exercise to enhance weight loss and improve blood pressure and cholesterol. Even 30 minutes a day of brisk exercise can have significant benefits.

Specific dietary changes often include restricting carbohydrates to no more than 50% of daily calorie intake, increasing fiber consumption (especially from fruits and vegetables), reducing the amount of red meat and poultry in the diet and restricting unhealthy fats.

Quitting smoking is another important treatment for metabolic syndrome, as smoking not only promotes heart disease but also increases insulin resistance. In some cases, medication therapies may also be used to help control high cholesterol and high blood pressure, improve insulin resistance and manage obesity.

PLATE 22

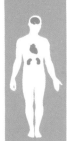

Understanding Diabetes

Glucose metabolism

After a meal, carbohydrates are converted to glucose by the digestive system. The glucose then enters the bloodstream. The pancreas responds to the rise in the blood glucose level by producing insulin and secreting it into the bloodstream. Insulin has several effects — it suppresses glucose production in the liver, it signals the liver to increase glucose uptake, and it allows glucose to enter cells from the bloodstream. As a result of these actions, blood glucose levels fall, insulin production ceases, and homeostasis is restored.

When the blood glucose level drops too far (such as after skipping a meal), the pancreas produces glucagon and secretes it into the bloodstream. Glucagon signals the liver to change glycogen into glucose and to release the glucose into the bloodstream. As blood glucose levels rise, glucagon production ceases, and homeostasis is restored.

Glucose

Insulin stimulates cells to take up glucose

Glucagon signals the liver to convert glycogen to glucose and release the glucose into the blood

Glucose   Glycogen

Liver

Pancreas

What is diabetes?

Diabetes is a disease characterized by a chronic imbalance in the blood glucose levels. There are two primary types of diabetes. Diabetes can strike at any age, although historically, young people normally fall victim because insulin production completely ceases. Those afflicted at later ages have some insulin production, but not enough to maintain a healthy blood glucose level. There are also two lesser-known types of diabetes. One affects women during pregnancy and is termed "gestational diabetes." It most often disappears or subsides substantially after the pregnancy ends. The fourth type of diabetes is the result of pancreatic disease, hormonal irregularities, or harmful drug interaction.

Insulin

Blood glucose level

Glucagon
Epinephrine cortisol
Human growth hormone

Cells use glucose as fuel

Glucose is converted to triglycerides and stored in fat (adipose tissues)

Function of insulin

Insulin, which is produced by the pancreas, facilitates the absorption of glucose into muscles for fuel. Glucose provides power to the body, but is kept under control by insulin. When the body acts normally, insulin bonds to the surface of cells and, as glucose travels throughout the body, glucose is able to penetrate the cell and be used effectively. Insulin determines how much glucose is produced by the liver and between meals. It does this by countering another hormone, glucagon, also produced by the pancreas. Glucagon sends a message to the liver to convert glycogen to glucose.

The liver takes up glucose, converts it into glycogen and stores it

Action of insulin

Type I

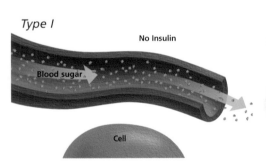

No Insulin

Blood sugar

Cell

Type I diabetes is less prevalent and occurs when there is a complete failure of the pancreas to produce insulin. It is considered an autoimmune disease. Type I diabetes occurs when antibodies produced by the body attack beta cells. Beta cells, which secrete insulin, are damaged over time and the cells eventually cease to produce the needed insulin. The absence of insulin allows ketones, normally a beneficial substance produced by the liver, to build up to abnormal levels, causing an acidosis (diabetic) coma.

Type II

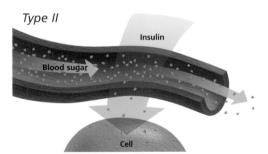

Insulin

Blood sugar

Cell

Type II diabetes occurs when the body resists the effects of insulin, or when there is a partial failure of the pancreas to produce insulin. Overweight people are often afflicted with this type of diabetes because their tissue becomes unable to respond to insulin and the pancreas is forced to produce more, but cannot meet the demand. The lack of insulin prevents glucose from entering the cells, so the body is not fully energized. This type of diabetes is normally diagnosed later in life as the continual strain on the pancreas leads to a decline of insulin production.

Normal

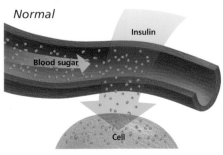

Insulin

Blood sugar

Cell

The interaction of glucose and insulin maintains a **normal level** of blood sugar and enables the body to perform daily activities.

Symptoms of diabetes

- Increased frequency of urination
- Unusually high desire for fluids
- Weight loss
- Blurred vision
- Weakness and fatigue
- Skin infections
- Complications that may include vascular disease and nerve damage

Health complications

Kidney damage

The kidney's ability to filter waste from the bloodstream is hindered by diabetes. High glucose levels, plus the common side effect of high blood pressure, damage the group of capillaries within the kidney called the glomeruli. A normal kidney filters waste and discharges it through the urine, allowing the necessary proteins to flow back through the body. Kidney damage, termed "nephropathy," is irreversible, leaving dialysis or a kidney transplant as the only two means to replace vital kidney processes once complete kidney failure occurs.

Narrowing of renal artery

Diseased kidney

Enlarged heart
Normal heart
Damaged heart tissue

Blocked coronary arteries

Vision problems

Vision problems are a common side effect of diabetes, specifically a condition known as retinopathy. In this eye complication, the small blood vessels that supply the retina with blood weaken and leak, damaging the retina and hindering its ability to transmit images to the brain. A more severe condition arises when fragile blood vessels grow into the vitreous humor (a jelly-like substance at the back of the eyeball) and rupture. Diabetics also have an increased risk for glaucoma and cataracts.

Retina

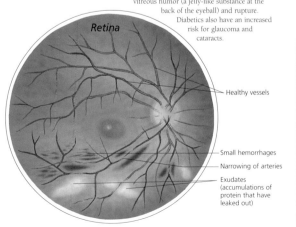

Healthy vessels

Small hemorrhages

Narrowing of arteries

Exudates (accumulations of protein that have leaked out)

Heart disease

Atherosclerosis, or narrowing of the arteries, may cause circulation to deteriorate in the coronary arteries. This leads to an increased possibility of angina, pain caused by a reduced blood flow to the heart, or heart attack. Strokes are also more prevalent in diabetics, as arteries to the brain are also affected by reduced blood flow.

Treatment and healthy lifestyle changes

Proper diabetes control depends on glucose levels. When glucose levels are too low, diabetics occasionally experience hypoglycemia, or low blood sugar. Hypoglycemia typically occurs when the insulin dosage exceeds the amount needed, such as between meals. The opposite condition is hyperglycemia, resulting when the body is not able to burn off sugars through physical activity. Both conditions occur often in diabetics because glucose levels controlled through medication cannot be as precisely regulated as through the body's natural mechanisms.

The successful treatment for diabetes, a non-curable disease, requires that patients maintain a healthy lifestyle through diet, medication and exercise. Here are a few suggestions:

1) Monitor blood glucose levels. Seek the advice of a doctor or nurse as to the type (blood or urine) and the frequency of tests required.

2) Eat regularly and do not skip meals. This advice is very important to maintain proper blood glucose levels. The amount of food eaten must be balanced with the amount of energy expended. If the patient is taking insulin, regular consultation with a dietician or nurse is recommended to help coordinate the timing of injections with meals.

3) Choose the right foods. Balance starchy, high-fiber foods with vegetables, fruits, and proteins. Avoid sweets and high-fat foods. Limit salt intake.

4) Limit or avoid alcohol. For patients on medication, whether orally or by injection, alcohol can lead to a hypoglycemic attack.

5) Exercise regularly.

6) Maintain ideal body weight. Lose weight if necessary by eating a well-balanced diet. Avoid fad diets.

7) Take medication as prescribed.

Nerve damage

Diabetics' higher glucose levels make them more susceptible to nerve damage. The most common form is peripheral neuropathy, which causes limbs to tingle as a result of the reduced function of sensory nerves. Peripheral neuropathy develops slowly and creates numbness and pain in the hands and legs. Other forms of nerve damage may also affect the digestive tract, bladder and other internal organs.

PLATE 23

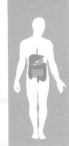

Understanding Cholesterol

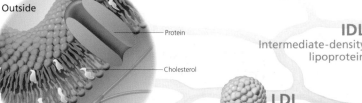

Cell membrane

Outside

- Protein
- Cholesterol

Inside

How cholesterol travels

High-density lipoproteins carry excess cholesterol away from cells for reprocessing in the liver or elimination through the digestive system. This mechanism protects against high cholesterol as well as atherosclerosis or "hardening of the arteries." When HDL levels are too low, less cholesterol is removed from the tissues and cholesterol levels increase.

Low-density lipoproteins carry cholesterol produced in the liver to tissues throughout the body. High concentrations of LDL are a leading factor in the development of atherosclerosis.

Very low-density lipoproteins, consisting primarily of cholesterol with little protein, also carry cholesterol to the body's tissues and can deposit cholesterol on blood vessel walls.

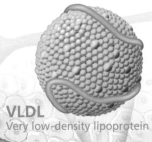

IDL
Intermediate-density lipoprotein

LDL
Low-density lipoprotein

VLDL
Very low-density lipoprotein

HDL

HDL

HDL
High-density lipoprotein

What is cholesterol?

Cholesterol is a natural, fat-like substance that is indispensable to the human body. It is a key component of cells, helping to maintain the stability and fluidity of **cell membranes**. It is utilized abundantly in the liver to produce **cholic acid**, which forms the bile salts necessary for **fat digestion**. Cholesterol is also necessary for the formation of hormones such as **estrogen** and **testosterone**. Significant amounts of cholesterol are used in the skin to synthesize **Vitamin D** and to help control **water evaporation** through the pores.

The body's cholesterol supply comes from two sources. It is primarily manufactured in the **liver**, along with several other organs in the body. It is also ingested through food, particularly **eggs**, **red meat**, and **dairy products** high in cholesterol content.

What does "high cholesterol" mean?

Blood cholesterol tests measure the amount of cholesterol bound to **lipoproteins**, fat-protein complexes that carry fats through the bloodstream. A diagnosis of high cholesterol or **hypercholesterolemia** indicates total cholesterol levels of 240 mg/dL or above (*see chart below*). More specifically, it indicates unhealthy levels of **low-density lipoproteins (LDL)**, **high-density lipoproteins (HDL)**, and/or **triglycerides**. High cholesterol caused by any of these factors increases the risk of **coronary artery disease** and potential **heart attack**.

High cholesterol is often thought of as an excess amount of LDL ("bad") cholesterol. However, an abnormally low HDL ("good") cholesterol level is an equally important risk factor for heart disease. Elevated triglyceride levels are also associated with increased risk, especially in combination with obesity and other factors.

Cholesterol guidelines (*see chart below*) are used to identify appropriate cholesterol levels for different individuals. Another valuable tool for predicting coronary artery disease is a **risk ratio**. This calculation measures the ratio of one form of cholesterol to another by dividing total cholesterol by either the HDL or LDL level.

- Optimal risk ratio – 3:5
- Average risk ratio – 4:5
- Increased risk ratio – 5:1

Chylomicron lipoprotein

Return path for approximately 50% of IDLs

Endogenous pathway

Most of the cholesterol used by the body is **endogenous**, formed in the body's cells. This process primarily involves **high-density lipoproteins (HDL)**, which transport endogenous cholesterol synthesized in the intestines and other organs.

- **VLDL** secreted in the liver is carried to muscle and adipose tissue
- VLDL is converted to **LDL**
- Metabolism of LDL occurs in liver and other cells
- HDL picks up excess cholesterol in the cells (including **artery walls**) and returns it to the **liver** for disposal

Chylomicron fragments

Liver

Gallbladder

Bile duct

The balance of HDL and LDL is largely determined by the flow of cholesterol between the body's cells and the liver.

Duodenum

Exogenous pathway

Exogenous cholesterol is absorbed by the body through the gastrointestinal tract. The transportation of exogenous cholesterol is primarily performed by **low-density lipoproteins (LDL)**, which contain most of the body's total cholesterol.

- **Chylomicrons** in the intestinal wall absorb triglycerides and cholesterol from the diet
- Chylomicrons are hydrolyzed in the **intestinal lymphatic** system
- The triglyceride content of chylomicrons is removed by **lipoprotein lipase**
- Fatty acids are released into **muscle** and **adipose tissue**

What is a lipoprotein?

Lipoproteins are spherical complexes that carry fat molecules through the blood stream. They consist of a water-soluble outer protein shell, a central phospholipid layer, and an inner cholesterol or triglyceride core. Lipoproteins are categorized by their **size** and **density**.

- The smallest lipoproteins carry **cholesterol** (LDL and HDL)
- The largest lipoproteins carry **triglycerides**, the leading source of fat in the diet and body tissues
- Large lipoprotein complexes include **very low-density lipoproteins (VLDL)** and **chylomicrons**, short-lived compounds that carry dietary cholesterol and triglycerides from the small intestines to the tissues after eating.

Cholesterol limits

Current guidelines published by the National Cholesterol Education Program (NCEP) recommend **periodic cholesterol testing** in all adults beginning at age 20.

- Adults with normal cholesterol levels require retesting every 5 years
- Patients being treated for high cholesterol should be retested every 2 to 6 months
- Selective screening should be conducted for children with inherited risks of high cholesterol

The NCEP advocates testing for a **total lipoprotein profile**. Current recommendations for total cholesterol, LDL, HDL, and triglyceride levels are listed below:

Total Cholesterol (mg/dL)	HDL Cholesterol (mg/dL)
Desirable: <200	Low: <40
Borderline high: 200-239	High: >60
High: >240	

LDL Cholesterol (mg/dL)	Serum Triglycerides (mg/dL)
Optimal: <100	Normal: <150
Near/above optimal: 100-129	Borderline high: 150-199
Borderline high: 130-159	High: 200-499
High: 160-189	Very high: >500
Very high: >190	

Reabsorption

Dietary intake

Epithelial cells in the small intestine

Reabsorption and elimination

Both ingested and manufactured cholesterol are converted to **bile** in the liver and recirculated many times in the body. Bile enters the intestine via the liver and **bile duct**. After digestion, a high percentage of secreted cholesterol and the bile salts are reabsorbed from the **large intestine** and removed from the blood by the liver. They are then excreted again into bile. Cholesterol that is not recycled during absorption is eliminated as waste.

Elimination through waste

Plaque
Ruptured plaque
Blood clot
Embolus

Causes and treatment of high cholesterol

Causes
High cholesterol is caused by a number of factors that can be controlled to prevent or reduce the risk of heart disease.

High saturated fat and cholesterol intake increase total blood cholesterol by increasing production of cholesterol in the liver and slowing cholesterol elimination from the body.

Being overweight elevates cholesterol levels and increases the risk of heart disease.

A sedentary lifestyle increases LDL levels and decreases protective levels of HDL.

Smoking also increases heart disease risks by reducing protective HDL.

Age, gender and heredity also play a role in elevated cholesterol. These factors can make cholesterol levels more difficult to control.

Treatment
Lowering cholesterol can require a combination of diet changes, increased exercise, and medication.

Dietary modification is the most important step in aggressively treating high cholesterol. Recommendations include:
- a maximum 7% daily dietary intake of saturated fats
- replacing saturated fats with unsaturated fats such as olive or canola oil
- a maximum 200 mg/day of cholesterol intake
- increased consumption of fiber-rich foods including whole grains and fruits and vegetables

Regular physical activity is also essential to:
- lower LDL levels
- increase HDL levels
- promote weight loss
- reduce the risk of atherosclerosis

Medication therapy is used to reduce cholesterol when diet and exercise are not sufficient. Lipid-lowering drugs can:
- improve the balance of HDL and LDL
- reduce serum triglyceride levels

Normal artery

Artery with plaque

What is atherosclerosis?

Atherosclerosis is the gradual buildup of plaque in the arteries, caused primarily by **low-density lipoprotein (LDL)** deposited inside the vessel walls. Localized plaques or atheromas made up of fats and cholesterol thicken and eventually protrude into the artery. While small **atheromas** often remain soft, older atheromas may become larger and develop fibrous calcium deposits on the surface. During progression of the disease, arteries become increasingly calcified and inelastic, reducing or blocking blood flow and preventing oxygen-rich blood from reaching the heart. Atheromas present an additional danger if they become sites for blood clots, which may rupture and result in a heart attack.

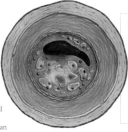

Complete blockage

Progression of plaque development

- Oxidized low-density lipoproteins initiate endothelial cell injury
- Fatty streaks consisting of lipid-filled macrophages and lymphocytes appear
- Layers of macrophages and smooth muscle are present
- Lesions or fibrous plaques develop over accumulated lipids and debris, protruding into the artery

PLATE 24

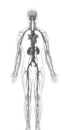

The Effects of Alcohol

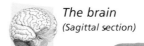
The brain
(Sagittal section)

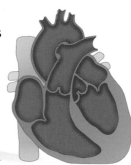

- Striatum
- Nucleus accumbens
- Prefrontal cortex
- Substantia nigra
- Ventral tegmental area

What is alcohol?

Alcoholic beverages contain **ethanol**, a clear, thin, odorless liquid created by the fermentation of fruit or grain mixtures (wine and beer) or the distillation of fermented fruit or grain mixtures (whiskey, gin, vodka and rum). The exact concentration of ethanol varies according to the type of beverage. On average, beer is 4.5 percent ethanol; wine is 11 percent ethanol; and distilled spirits range from 40 to 95 percent ethanol. Pure alcohol should never be consumed, as it quickly produces effects that can become fatal.

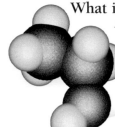

Ethanol
C_2H_6O

How alcohol affects the body

Alcohol affects virtually every part of the body. In the gastrointestinal system, alcohol irritates the linings of the esophagus and stomach, triggers the secretion of acid and histamine, and can cause vomiting. Over time, alcohol use can lead to gastritis or ulcers. Alcohol consumption also increases blood flow to the skin, resulting in lost body heat, while at the same time decreasing blood flow to the muscles. Brain and liver cells are directly affected by alcohol, even with occasional drinking.

Long-term effects of heavy drinking include more serious complications, such as:

- Liver enlargement and damage such as alcoholic hepatitis and cirrhosis
- High blood pressure, stroke, irregular heartbeat and heart damage or disease
- Kidney failure resulting from chronic alcohol-induced diuresis
- Increased risk of mouth, larynx, liver and gastrointestinal cancers
- Greater incidence of pneumonia and acute respiratory distress syndrome (ARDS)
- Dietary deficiencies of essential nutrients such as iron, folic acid, and thiamine, which may lead to nerve damage
- Impairment of memory, thinking and concentration skills
- Death of brain cells and reduced brain mass
- Higher risk of injury from falls or accidents
- Decreased production of sex hormones
- Personality changes and other emotional and behavioral problems, including anxiety or depression

Acute overdoses of alcohol, also known as alcohol poisoning, produce symptoms including nausea and vomiting, loss of consciousness, depressed respiration, lack of reflexes, and in severe cases, coma. Blood alcohol concentrations above .40–.50 are considered lethal and may be fatal if not treated immediately.

Nervous system effects

Synaptic knob or axon terminal of presynaptic neuron

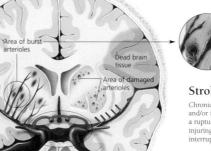

- Mitochondria
- Synaptic vesicles
- Neurotransmitter molecules
- Synaptic cleft
- Receptor sites
- Ions
- Postsynaptic cell

Dopamine pathways

The dopamine pathway is one component of the brain reward system. This pathway may also be involved in an ethanol reinforcement effect.

Alcohol and neurotransmitters

Alcohol directly affects the function of important chemical messengers in the brain known as neurotransmitters. These highly specialized chemicals stimulate nerve impulses from one neuron to another neuron, muscle or gland, either inhibiting or activating neural impulses. Normal levels of neurotransmitters, such as dopamine, serotonin, opiate neuropeptides, GABA (a major inhibitory transmitter) and glutamate receptors are negatively altered by alcohol consumption.

Cardiovascular effects

Damage to the heart

Cardiomyopathy is a disease of the heart muscle. The muscle fibers are damaged and the heart chamber walls are weakened. To compensate for this injury the chambers of the heart enlarge. The function of the heart is impaired, resulting in inadequate blood flow to the body's organs and tissues. Heart rhythm can be disturbed, with resulting heartbeat irregularities, or arrhythmias. About one-third of cardiomyopathy cases are from excessive alcohol consumption. Alcoholic cardiomyopathy can eventually lead to heart failure.

Normal heart

Heart with cardiomyopathy
- *Damaged muscle fibers*
- *Weakened heart chamber walls*
- *Enlarged heart chambers*

Fetal alcohol syndrome

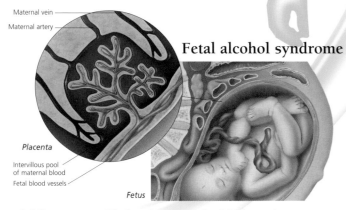

- Maternal vein
- Maternal artery
- *Placenta*
- Intervillous pool of maternal blood
- Fetal blood vessels
- *Fetus*

Alcohol in a pregnant woman's bloodstream is passed directly through the placenta and into the developing baby's bloodstream. High alcohol consumption by a pregnant mother can cause fetal alcohol syndrome, which is associated with:

- Mental retardation and developmental delays
- Small body size, slow growth and poor coordination
- Heart defects
- Hearing, vision and dental defects
- Facial abnormalities
- Behavioral problems including hyperactivity and limited attention span

Drinking alcohol during pregnancy also increases the risks of miscarriage, stillbirth and low birth weight.

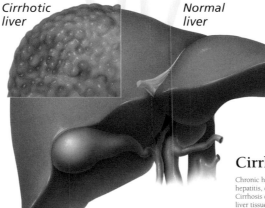

- Area of burst arterioles
- Dead brain tissue
- Area of damaged arterioles
- Area of burst arterioles
- Circle of Willis

Stroke

Chronic heavy drinking and binge drinking may result in a hemorrhagic and/or ischemic stroke. A hemorrhagic stroke occurs when blood from a ruptured vessel accumulates and compresses surrounding brain tissue, injuring cells and interfering with brain function. The leaking vessel also interrupts oxygen flow to the brain.

Brain in cross section

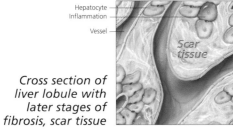

- Hepatocyte
- Inflammation
- Vessel
- *Scar tissue*

Cross section of liver lobule with later stages of fibrosis, scar tissue

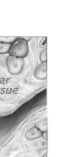

Cirrhotic liver

Normal liver

Cirrhosis of the liver

Chronic heavy drinking can cause alcoholic hepatitis, cirrhosis or complete liver failure. Cirrhosis develops when a significant portion of liver tissue is progressively and irreversibly destroyed by alcohol abuse.

Kidney effects

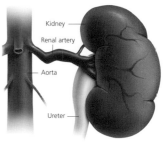

- Kidney
- Renal artery
- Aorta
- Ureter

The kidneys have several functions, including elimination of cellular waste products, regulation of fluid and electrolyte volumes and concentrations, and production of hormones. Alcohol can compromise the functioning of the kidneys in several ways. Through its ability to increase urine volume, alcohol alters the body's fluid level, which changes the electrolyte balance. The effects of this imbalance vary, but can include dehydration and impaired mental activity. Brain cells, particularly neurons, are highly affected by the electrolyte balance. Alcohol also disrupts the hormonal regulation of the kidney through changes in plasma volume and blood pressure. Impairment of liver function from alcohol can result in compromised kidney function, such as impaired fluid handling.

Intoxication levels

The degree of alcohol intoxication depends on multiple factors, including body size, the amount and rate of alcohol consumption, the rate of absorption (influenced by the presence or absence of food in the stomach), how the body metabolizes alcohol, genetics and previous drinking experience. As a general rule, alcohol that is consumed slowly (7 grams per hour or approximately 1.5 ounces of 80% proof distilled spirits) will not accumulate in the body or result in intoxication.

BAC*	Effects
.01 – .05 %	Feelings of relaxation, lowered inhibitions
.05 – .07 %	Impairment begins; loss of coordination, reflexes and muscle control; loss of self-control and driving capability
.08 – .10 %	Legally drunk in almost all states and the District of Columbia
.10 – .15 %	Loss of balance, impaired body coordination and slightly slurred speech
.15 – .25 %	Slurred speech, difficulty walking, confusion, loss of perception, vision problems
.25 – .40 %	Most people are in a state of stupor; loss of consciousness, some may die
.40 – .50 + %	Most people are unconscious, breathing shuts off; coma and death are likely

*Approximate Blood Alcohol Concentration

What is alcoholism?

Alcoholism or alcohol dependence is a disease that is usually chronic and progressive and frequently fatal. Symptoms of alcoholism include:

- Emotional and physical dependence on alcohol
- Blackouts and hangovers
- Alcohol-related health problems
- Unpleasant withdrawal symptoms
- Lack of control over the amount or frequency of drinking
- Preoccupation with drinking
- Personality changes and emotional and psychiatric difficulties

Alcohol dependence can take many forms, ranging from occasional drinking to chronic heavy drinking or binge drinking. Most people with alcohol dependence continue to drink even if alcohol is affecting their physical or mental health. Many alcoholics need increasing amounts of alcohol to become intoxicated and experience severe withdrawal symptoms during periods of abstinence. They may also have poor nutrition, gastrointestinal problems, numbness or weakness in the legs and hands, and problems with balance.

Treatment

The first step in treatment is acknowledgement of a drinking problem and a decision to stop drinking. Depending on the severity of the disease, either inpatient or outpatient detoxification may be necessary to help the body reverse its dependence on alcohol. Medical treatment may also include tranquilizers, vitamin supplements and intravenous fluids. Drugs such as disulfiram and naltrexone are sometimes prescribed to reduce the craving for alcohol. Other important components of alcoholism treatment include long-term psychological counseling, self-help groups and counseling for family members.

PLATE 25